GW00500211

# PHARMACY HISTORY

### A Pictorial Record

Photographs from the Museum of the
Royal Pharmaceutical Society of Great Britain

Nigel Tallis and Kate Arnold-Forster

London
THE PHARMACEUTICAL PRESS
1991

Copies of this book may be obtained through any good bookseller,
or in any case of difficulty, direct from the publisher or the publisher's agents:

The Pharmaceutical Press
(Publications division of the Royal Pharmaceutical Society of Great Britain)
1 Lambeth High Street
London  SE1 7JN
England

*Australia*
The Australian Pharmaceutical Publishing Co. Ltd.
40 Burwood Road, Hawthorn, Victoria 3122 *and*
Pharmaceutical Society of Australia
Pharmaceutical House, P.O. Box 21, Curtin ACT 2605

*Germany, Austria, Switzerland*
Deutscher Apotheker Verlag
Birkenwaldstrasse 44, D-7000 Stuttgart 1

*India*
Arnold Publishers (India) Pte. Ltd.
AB/9 Safdarjung Enclave, New Delhi 110029

*Japan*
Maruzen Co. Ltd.
3-10 Nihonbashi 2-chome, Chuo-ku, Tokyo 103

*New Zealand*
The Pharmaceutical Society of New Zealand
124 Dixon Street, P.O. Box 11-640, Wellington

*USA*
Rittenhouse Book Distributors Inc.
511 Feheley Drive, King of Prussia, Pennsylvania 19406

All copy photography by Rod Tidnam
Designed and typeset by Baseline Creative Ltd., Bath BA2 3DZ, and printed and bound by The Bath Press, Bath BA2 3BL

**British Library Cataloguing in Publication Data**
Tallis, Nigel
Pharmacy History : a pictorial record.
1. Great Britain. Pharmacy, history
I. Title  II. Arnold-Forster, Kate
362. 17820941

ISBN 0-85369-241-6

# CONTENTS

Introduction  1
The Society's House  4
Portraits  11
Jacob Bell Memorial Scholars  19
Benevolent Fund  21
Pharmacy Education and Schools of Pharmacy  22
Conferences and Meetings  35
Pharmacy Premises  46
Social Setting  78
Pharmacy Raw Materials and Production  82

Illustrations Index  89
Photographer Index  92

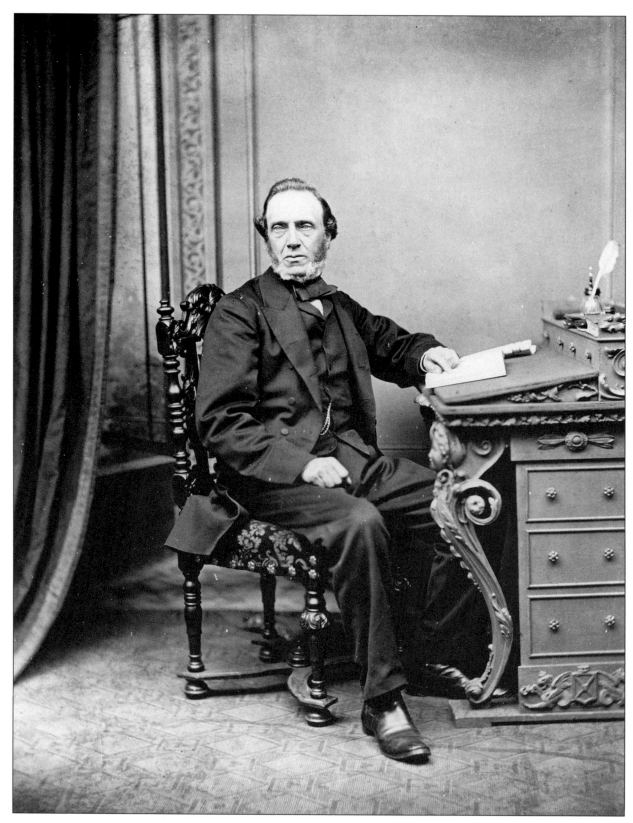

Plate 1.
"One of Mr Swan's earliest carbon prints". John Mawson, 1863.

# INTRODUCTION

*"Dr Pereira informs me you have got a new trick –
something that is done in the dark
I forget the name of it but I think it is called horoography"*

*Jacob Bell* [1]

In 1986 the Museum of the Royal Pharmaceutical Society of Great Britain initiated a project to document and conserve its historical photographs as a pilot scheme for the retrospective documentation of the entire museum collection. The Society's photographic collection is a small but growing archive of some 12,000 items, consisting of over 8,000 different photographic images, both negative and positive, colour and monochrome. The variety of formats represented in the collection reflects the considerable diversity of photographic processes evolved in 150 years of development, and includes daguerreotypes, gelatin, albumen and carbon prints, collodion and gelatin glass plate negatives, lantern slides, and colour transparencies. During the course of the cataloguing project it became clear that the collection contained some fine examples of work produced by several distinguished early photographers, while other images highlighted the significant contributions made by chemists and druggists to the development of photography - as illustrated by the extremely rare experimental example of Sir Joseph Wilson Swan's improved carbon process (pl. 1).

The overwhelming majority of these images are original and unique and greatly augment the Society's other archives to form a significant, and in many ways unrivalled, historical record. It is only comparatively recently that the true value of photographic images as an historical resource has become fully appreciated. The Society's collection not only illustrates the great changes in all aspects of pharmacy in Britain over the previous 140 years, but also provides abundant details of costume,

topography, technology, and other wider social historical developments.

The Pharmaceutical Society of Great Britain was formally established on 15 April 1841. This was less than two years after the public announcement of the first practical commercial photographic process in August 1839, and within a month of the opening in London of Europe's first professional photographic studio, that of Richard Beard at the Royal Polytechnic Institution, on 23 March 1841. Many pharmaceutical businesses profited through photography in the supply of both chemicals, for which they were a natural and ready source, and apparatus for the new invention. Others specialised in photography,

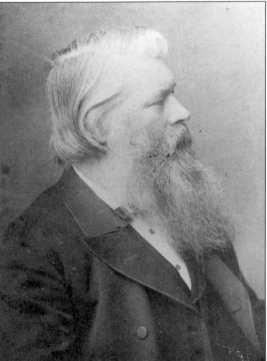

Plate 2.
Sir Joseph Wilson Swan, as president of the Newcastle-on-Tyne and Northern Counties Photographic Association, 1881.

even to the extent of improving and inventing new processes. Of these, the firm of John Mawson (1813-1867) and Joseph, later Sir Joseph, Wilson Swan FRS (1828-1914) of Newcastle-upon-Tyne was only the most strikingly successful (pl. 2). Swan, whose many inventions included the carbon filament electric light and the first portable miners' electric safety lamp, was to remark in later life concerning his hard apprenticeship with Hudson & Osbaldiston in Sunderland, that it was "not a quite unalloyed pleasure for me to look back to the days of my first contact with pharmacy".[2] However, his later partnership with Mawson led to many significant and successful advances in photography, particularly his brands of photographic collodion ("Mawson's Collodion" of 1854) for the wet collodion process, his gelatin dry plates ("Swan's Plates" of 1876), and especially Swan's improved carbon process perfected by 1866.

Pharmacists supplied materials, processing, and often the entire range of photographic apparatus to the rapidly increasing number of amateur photographers. The designation of "photographic chemist" became widespread in the later nineteenth century, and is of course still in evidence. This ready and extensive adjunct to other more specialist photographic suppliers must have played a considerable part in the popularisation of photography. Something of a country pharmacist's predicament in dealing with this new craze can be judged from an article in *The Chemist and Druggist* for 1861:

"Photography has spread so wonderfully through the length and breadth of the land that there is scarcely a hamlet or village too small or insignificant not to be visited at least occasionally by some of the votaries of the art. The quiet chemists of the picturesque townlets are now and then frightened from their propriety by the apparition of a mild gentleman in spectacles, with very black fingers and wristbands, who asks, in a very courteous, but excited manner, for a small quantity of pyrogallic acid, he having 'unfortunately left his bottle behind him' - or, if there is no artistic 'bit' in the neighbourhood, the questioner is very possibly a mountebank-looking party, in a velveteen coat, with no shirt collar, a closely shaven beard, and curly black hair, who asks for 'two hounces of postiv clodion, nooly mixed'. The poor chemist is aghast, he looks furtively in his *Pharm. Lond.* for 1833 for pyrogallic acid, and finds nothing but gallic acid, which the mild gentleman politely tells him will not do. As for the 'postiv clodion', he supposes the man must mean collodion, and forthwith serves him with two ounces of it, in a fine ropy condition, which is shortly afterwards returned by the seedy 'professional', with a few observations not remarkable for their elegance, or their friendliness to the chemist's eyes. The poor amateur is obliged to go away disappointed of his view, and the 'professional' is prevented from taking a number of patent enamelled American ivory-type portraits of the Chloes and Strephons of the place, at 6d each, frame and glass included."[3]

Later in the nineteenth century picture postcards were a "most lucrative" sideline for pharmacists. John Cleworth of Manchester described issuing sets of printing-out paper postcards from his own negatives at 2d each:

"For the 2d cards I make a point of photographing every exciting event in the neighbourhood, which negatives I develop as quickly as possible...I print these on glossy Velox cards, and in about two hours postcards of the event are ready for sale. I have done well with local fires..."[4]

A marked interest in photography is also evident from the earliest days of the Pharmaceutical Society. In 1843, Jacob Bell (1810-1859), founder of the Pharmaceutical Society and owner and first editor of *The Pharmaceutical Journal* wrote, with his usual

disingenuous wit, the opening lines quoted at the head of this introduction to solicit an article by Henry Collen on the photographic process he called "Thermography". More significantly, an anonymous essay entitled "The Application of the Daguerreotype Process to the Arts", almost certainly by Bell, which appeared in *The Pharmaceutical Journal* in 1846, discusses the practical use of photographic images as an aid for making engravings from paintings.[5] In this short article, illustrated with an example of an engraving made from a daguerreotype of T.N.R. Morson's (1799-1874) laboratory, the author demonstrates considerable knowledge of the advantages and disadvantages of contemporary photography in relation to the traditional arts. This is particularly interesting in view of Jacob Bell's friend, William Powell Frith's (1819-1909) somewhat clandestine use of photography in the production of his paintings, and specifically for his famous and "vulgar" work *Derby Day*, 1856-1858. Bell had specially commissioned this immensely popular painting, which earned for the artist through the sale of copyright and rights to exhibition

the then amazing sum of £2,250 in addition to the purchase price of £1,500.

As the business advisor of his friend Sir Edwin Landseer RA (1802-1873), and several other artists, Bell was well aware of the large sums of money to be made through assigning the copyright for engravings of popular works, and he clearly appreciated the commercial possibilities of photography in speeding the lengthy process of copying.

Of other founder members of the Society, Peter Squire (1798-1884) harboured a lamentable taste for the worst kind of genre art photographs, which included "6 splendid photographs, Faith, Hope & Charity, War, Peace & Plenty". In 1864, his son Alexander Balmanno Squire (d. 1908) produced *An Atlas of Coloured Photographs of the Diseases of the Skin*. Of the hand tinted illustrations *The Lancet* commented:

"To use a common expression, the photograph 'is life itself', and disease has never been more faithfully represented by art than it has been here." [6]

The latest advances in photography were regularly demonstrated at the Society's annual *Conversazione* at its headquarters in Bloomsbury Square. In 1845, for example, daguerreotypes from Antoine Claudet (1797-1867) and a Mr Willat (possibly T. or R. Willats) were displayed together with other objects of pharmaceutical interest.[7] On 17 May 1864 Claudet demonstrated indoor and night-time photography using a magnesium flash (following a similar show at the Society of Arts), while at the same meeting were exhibited examples of Claudet's "Photosculptures", an improved photographic tent, a self-acting photographic plate-washer, and photographic prints from the Royal Exchange Portrait Company. [8] Improvements in photography were closely observed, and formulae for new processes were often given in the pharmaceutical press. In 1861, the recently established journal, *The Chemist and Druggist,* announced a policy of providing lists of "chemicals which ought to be kept by every one of our subscribers, who has not already a well filled photographic corner in his shop".[9]

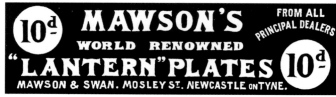

But despite the obvious and early interest in photography displayed by many leading members of the Pharmaceutical Society, funds do not appear to have been available for official or commemorative Society photographs. It was not until the early 1860s, when the Society apparently commissioned a series of high quality albumen prints recording the appearance of presidents, Council members and Society employees, that this interest was practically expressed. At the same time collections of *carte-de-visite* portrait photographs of beneficiaries of the Jacob Bell Memorial Scholarships and annuitants of the Society's Benevolent Fund were initiated. The former was assiduously maintained from 1861 to 1970, the latter from the 1870s until 1937. The Benevolent Fund archive was a particularly peculiar concept by modern standards: it now seems rather unreasonable that a beneficiary, acknowledged to be in severe financial difficulties, should be asked to provide a portrait photograph for the Society's archives! It is difficult to judge how far this policy may have been prompted by the theories then in vogue linking physiognomy and character, rather than by the mania for collecting *cartes-de-visite* in general.

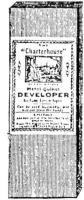

In the later nineteenth century the Society began to use photographs in promotional material for its School of Pharmacy and to provide mementoes for staff and students. Many of these images survive in the collection, as in some amusingly sycophantic Cabinet portraits of favourite members of staff (pl. 46) and numerous School group photographs from the 1860s to the late 1940s. Photographs of the Society's headquarters buildings in Bloomsbury Square began with a series taken after renovations to the building in 1883/4. Copies of these prints were mounted and framed for display in the library. Similar sets were produced in 1928 and 1932 which additionally illustrated the various activities of the Society. High quality photographs taken by members of staff, especially by Dr T.E. Wallis (1876-1973), amply document the building until the Society's departure for Lambeth in 1976. From the early years of this century, following the developments in photomechanical printing processes, a major part of the archive was derived from photographs used to illustrate *The Pharmaceutical Journal,* and a rather smaller number from *The Chemist and Druggist.* These include several original boards of camera-ready copy (pl. 123). Apart from these main areas of active, though irregular, collection the prime source of photographic material now held by the museum has been through private donations from members and pharmaceutical businesses. Representative of the latter are some unfortunately incomplete archives, notably from John Bell & Croyden (with groups from 1871, 1918, and 1933), Heppell & Co. (1912), S. Maw, Son & Sons (1920s), Steedman's (1920s-1950s), and Hooper's (1900-1960s). In the 1950s the Society's History of Pharmacy Committee, later to evolve into the British Society for the History of Pharmacy, made a determined and crucial effort to procure exterior photographs of those old-established and traditional pharmacies still surviving. Since 1986 the museum has in addition concentrated on the more under-represented areas of the archive, attempting in particular to acquire high quality images of contemporary, or near-contemporary pharmacy.

This book contains a small but representative selection of some of the earliest and most interesting images in the Society's specialist collection of historical photographs. It is the second publication to be based on material held in the Society's museum and recently catalogued as part of a computer database of the collections.[10] Although a considerable part of the photographic archive is naturally devoted to the Society's own history and activities, it is hoped that this publication will give some indication of the far wider scope of the collection. It is particularly appropriate, as the Royal Pharmaceutical Society reaches its sesquicentenary year, to be able to show to a wider audience these evocative images of pharmacy's past.

*Nigel Tallis*
*Kate Arnold-Forster*

1. *The Pharmaceutical Journal* 1933 **131** 296.

2. Reminiscences and Reflections, Address delivered at the opening of the session of the School of Pharmacy. *The Pharmaceutical Journal* 1903 **71** 477.

3. C.W. Quinn, Photographic Chemicals I, *The Chemist and Druggist* 1861 **2** 11.

4. Picture Postcards as a Side-Line, *The Chemist and Druggist* 1907 **70** 344.

5. *The Pharmaceutical Journal* 1846/7 **6** 251.

6. *The Lancet* 1864 **II** 182.

7. *The Pharmaceutical Journal* 1845/46 **5** 258.

8. *The Pharmaceutical Journal* 1863/64 **V** 604.

9. *The Chemist and Druggist* 1861 **2** 11. This policy was still evident at the end of the century, when details of the new Lumière "autochrome" colour plates were given "so that photographic-chemists will be able to meet promptly the demand for the solutions required".

10. The first, *The Bruising Apothecary. Images of Pharmacy and Medicine in Caricature,* was published in 1989 by the Pharmaceutical Press.

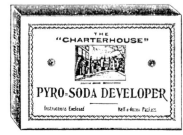

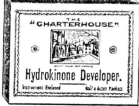

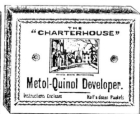

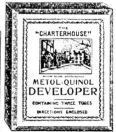

# THE SOCIETY'S HOUSE

It is slightly surprising, given the Society's justifiable pride in their headquarters, that the earliest photographs of the building at 17 Bloomsbury Square are the series of Martin & Sallnow albumen prints dating from as late as 1883/4 (pl.3). This seventeenth century building was flamboyantly remodelled by John Nash (1752-1835) in neo-classical style as a speculative venture in 1778; its original appearance may be seen preserved by the neighbouring buildings. The Society changed the building considerably during its long tenure from 1841 to 1976: adding the entrance porch and the pediments above the first floor windows, a whole new floor for laboratories in 1861, and having its name carved in large letters into the stucco below the architrave.

From 1883 the Society's house was regularly photographed, though because of the thick foliage of Bloomsbury Square, the best, indeed only, viewpoint looked towards the north-east corner of the building. The elevated view of c.1930 (pl. 4) is one of a very few variations on the theme; the new number 16, erected by the Society in 1890, can just be seen on the left.

The appearance of the original Council chamber on the second floor of Bloomsbury Square was not recorded, but in 1884 it had just been moved to a larger apartment (pl. 5). Note at this time the room was still only lighted by a single oil lamp while the rest of the building was lit by gas. Around the walls are portraits of Henry Deane (derived from the Maull print, pl. 26), Thomas Hyde Hills, Daniel Bell Hanbury, William Allen, and John Mackay.

By 1892 the Council room had moved yet again, at least the fifth move in 50 years, and the walls are quite crowded with portraits of worthies (pl. 6). The fine ceiling decoration was a legacy of Nash's earlier improvements.

In order to further the Society's ambitious educational aims, and to complement the School of Pharmacy, a museum and a library were established in 1842. The museum grew rapidly and soon moved to two large rooms by the entrance on the ground floor which it occupied until 1976. Its herbarium and important and exotic collections of materia medica proved an irresistible attraction for photographers, and visually it is very well documented. By 1883/4 the museum was lighted with gas lamps, and had fine modern showcases and cabinets to display the collections (pl. 7).

In 1928, and to an even greater extent after 1932, all the Society's many activities were recorded by two series of photographs for which the original full-plate glass negatives still exist. Although they are posed, in the sense that they are not spontaneous snapshots, the locations were evidently not tidied beforehand. Additionally, the staff were photographed at work, and the working environment was therefore recorded in exceptional detail. As can be seen compared with the staff group of 1898 (pl. 13) by 1937 (pl. 16) the office staff was considerably larger, and many were female.

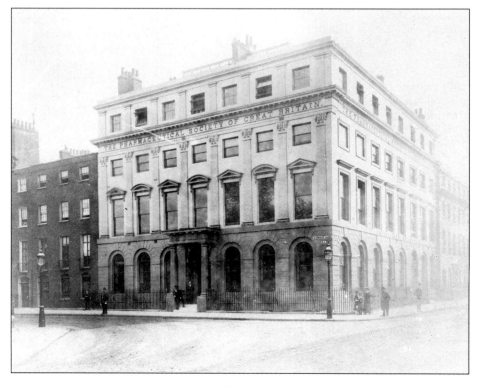

Plate 3.
Headquarters of the Pharmaceutical Society of Great Britain 1841-1976,
17 Bloomsbury Square, London, 1883/4.

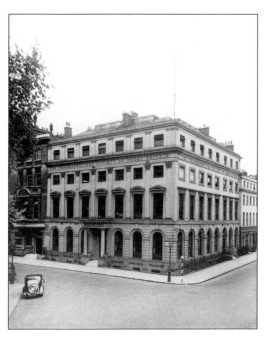

Plate 4.
The Pharmaceutical Society's house in the 1930s.

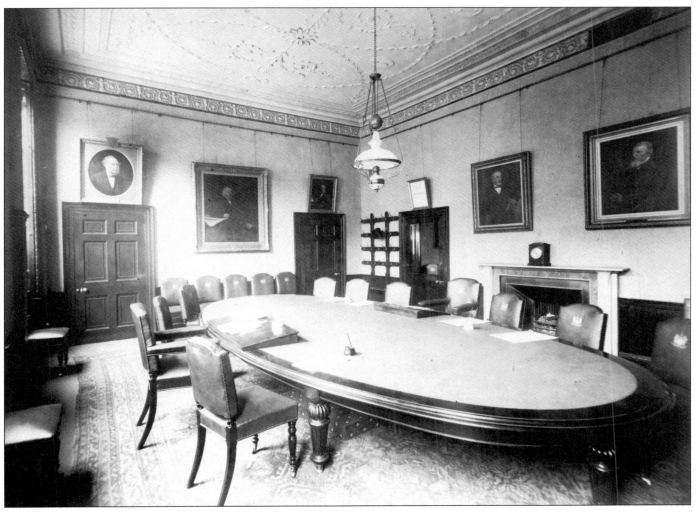

Plate 5.
The Council chamber, second floor of 17 Bloomsbury Square, 1883/4.

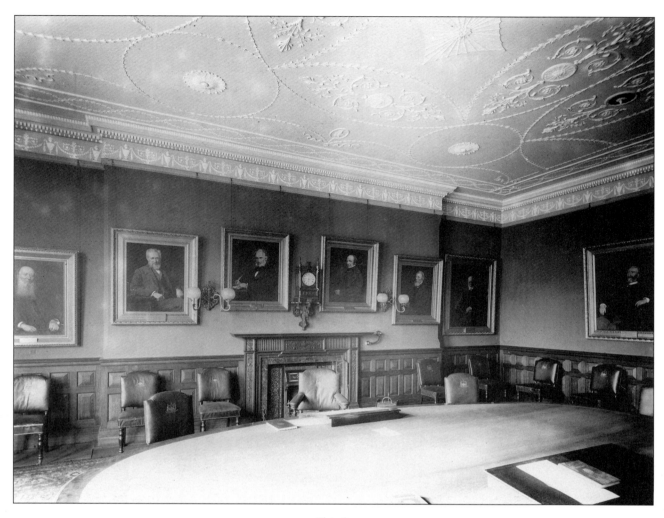

Plate 6.
The Council chamber, 17 Bloomsbury Square, 1892.

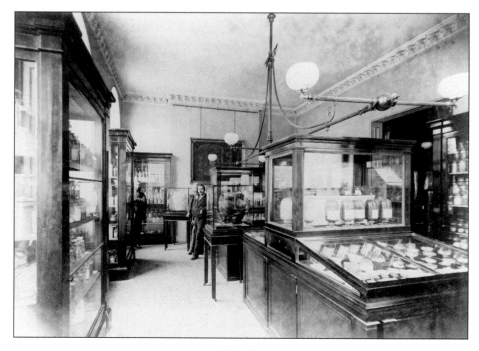

Plate 7.
The "Chemistry Museum", ground floor of 17 Bloomsbury Square, 1883/4.

7

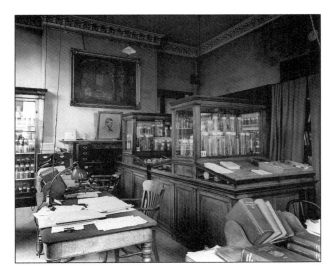

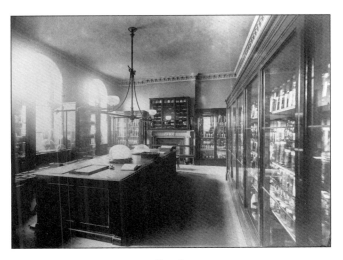

Plate 8.
The same view nearly 60 years later, 29 November 1937.

Plate 9.
The museum, 17 Bloomsbury Square, 1883/4.

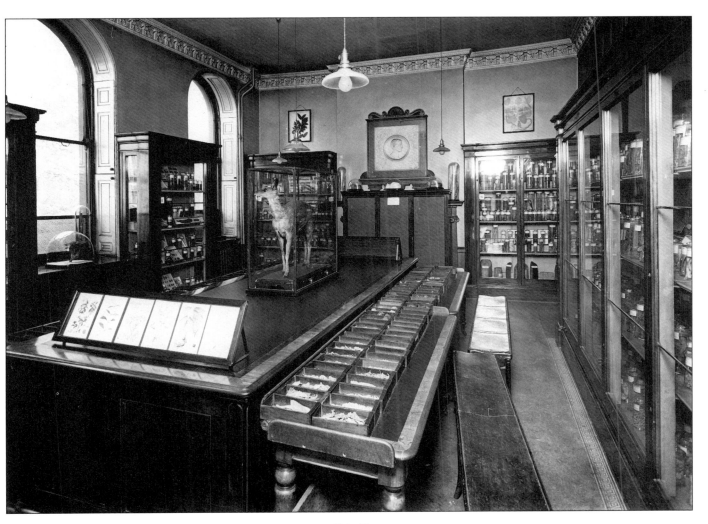

Plate 10.
The museum, 17 Bloomsbury Square, 1931.

8

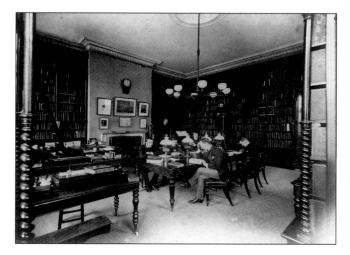

Plate 11.
The library, and readers, 17 Bloomsbury Square, 1883/4.

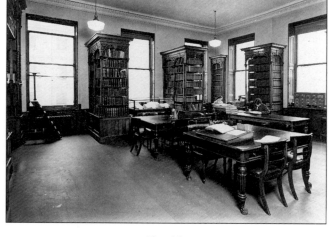

Plate 12.
Library, 17 Bloomsbury Square, 1928.

The library quickly expanded to take up two rooms on the first floor. The ornate bookcases were purchased secondhand from the 1863 International Exhibition.

In 1905, pressure of space at Bloomsbury Square was such that the hall and waiting room of the offices of *The Pharmaceutical Journal* were situated in the passageway of 72 Great Russell Street.

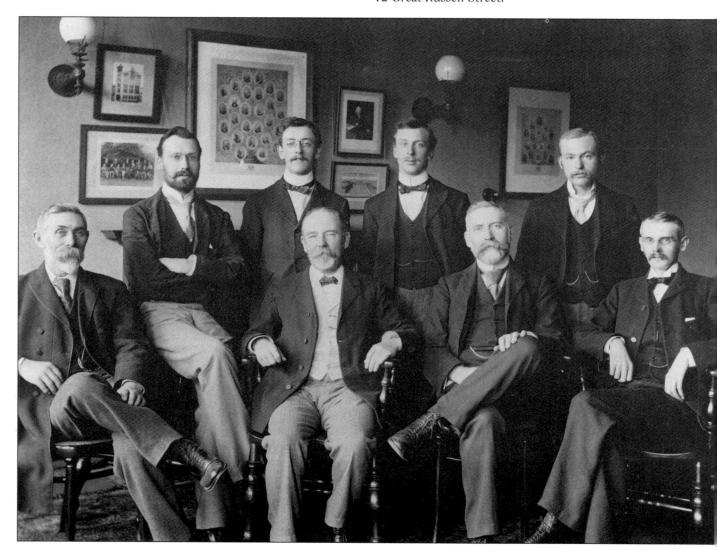

Plate 13.
The office staff, 1898.

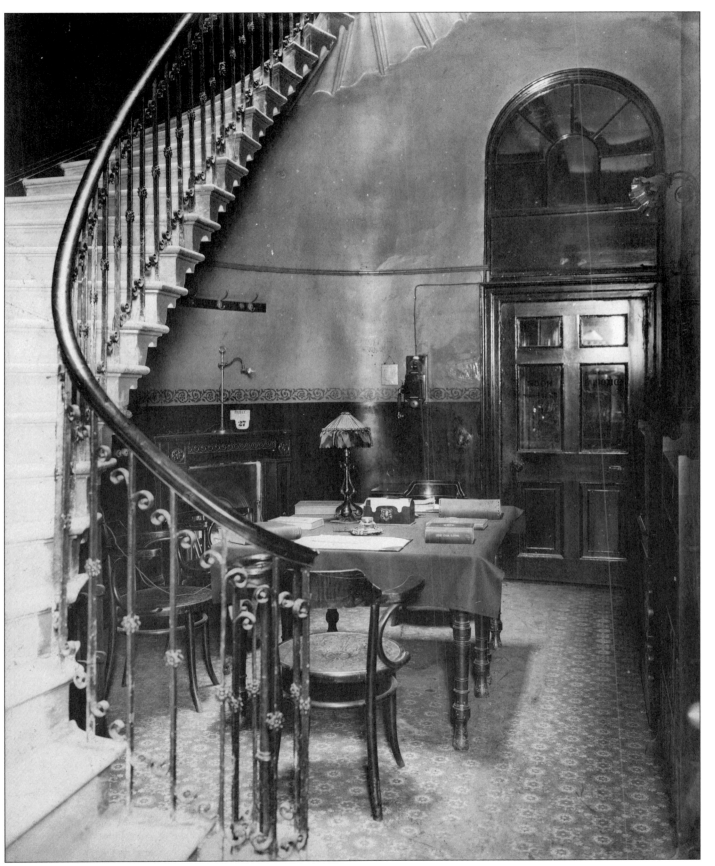

Plate 14.
Passage in 72 Great Russell Street, 1905, the *Pharmaceutical Journal's* waiting room.

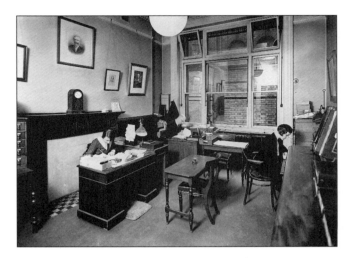

Plate 15.
Law department, ground floor, 16 Bloomsbury Square, October 1931.

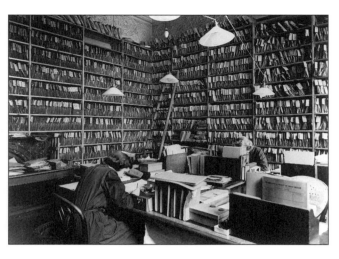

Plate 16.
Registry, 17 Bloomsbury Square, 1937.

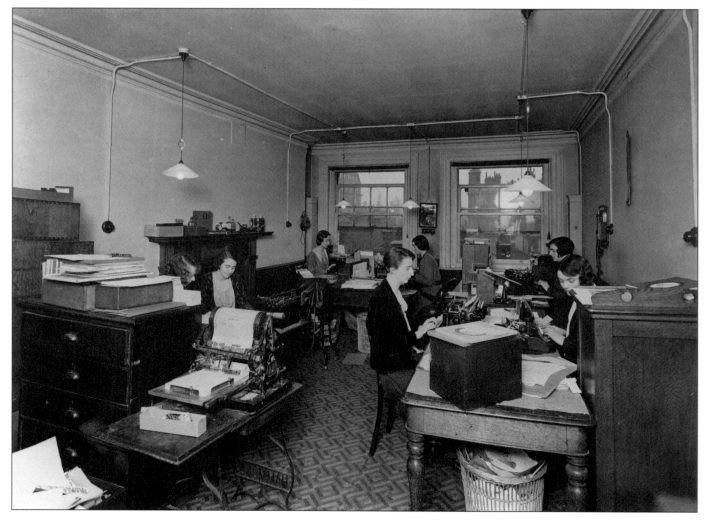

Plate 17.
Typists room on the third floor at the back of 16 Bloomsbury Square, 1931.

# PORTRAITS

The Society's collection of portraits is an instructive and often entertaining mix of public and private images. The earliest and finest portraits now in the collection are, as one might expect, photographs of the ubiquitous Jacob Bell. One is an original daguerreotype by J.E. Mayall of c.1852 (pl. 19), but the other, probably earlier example of the 1840s, possibly by Richard Beard, survives only as an albumen copy print made by Barrauds from a daguerreotype for the Society's anniversary celebrations of 1891 (pl. 18). A third daguerreotype, definitely by Beard and very similar to the Mayall version, is attested from an engraving in *The Illustrated London News* of 31 May 1851.

Some of the most interesting and characterful portraits in the collection are the personal and often humorous *carte-de-visite* portraits from a small album, probably the collection of Thomas Hyde Hills or Elias Bremridge. These photographs are frequently in marked contrast to the contemporary but rather stiff and stilted full-plate "official" Maull prints of many of the same subjects. The *cartes* represent the work of a wonderful variety of studios. These range from famous continental portraitists like Gaspard Felix Tournachon, "Nadar" (1820-1910), or the large metropolitan studios of J.E. Mayall (1810-1901), or Antoine Claudet (1797-1867), to small provincial photographers such as J.C. Brewer "Artist & Photographer" and J. Simpson. The capabilities of different studios varied greatly, and in many cases it might be observed that the actual choice of photographer is a rather better guide to the character of the subject than the final image.

In contrast to the *cartes,* the Maull pictures are severely formal portraits, and many were evidently framed for display at 17 Bloomsbury Square. They are the typical products of a reliable but uninspired commercial photographer and depict a selection of personalities from the Society's early years. Some, for example the prints of T.N.R. Morson and Henry Deane, were to be the basis for later oil portraits now in the Society's collection. This series

of images was most probably inspired by the Literary and Scientific Portrait Club, initiated by J.S. Bowerbank in 1854, which sold portrait prints by subscription. These Maull & Polyblank photographs had included portraits of Jacob Bell, T.N.R. Morson, Henry Deane and Peter Squire. The Society's prints, which also include portraits of Morson, Deane, and Squire, were produced by the same company but rather later, and were probably taken between 1865 and the early 1870s. At this time a number of firms were issuing commemorative portrait photographs of eminent medical personalities. For example, in 1864 Moira & Haigh published albums of portraits showing the medical staff of London's hospitals and Fellows of the College of Physicians,[11] and in the same year G.R. Fitt commenced a rival series of photographs of members of the Medical Council.[12]

The earliest Society portraits are all of individuals, and group photographs are not common until the 1900s, when the number of studio portraits declines markedly. The Council was apparently not photographed together until 1893, and this only became a fairly regular practice in the 1930s. There are a few studio portraits of local associations and branches, such as the members of the Bristol Pharmaceutical Association, c.1890, who were obviously too many for the photographer's backdrop (pl.37)!

Thomas Hyde Hills (1815-1891), was bequeathed the business of John Bell & Co. by his close friend Jacob Bell. Like Bell he was a friend to many artists, and succeeded Bell as Landseer's agent. He had been apprenticed in Brighton to a past apprentice of John Bell & Co., which business he himself joined in 1837 as a junior assistant. Hills was elected to the Council of the Society in 1860, was vice-president from 1863 to 1868, treasurer from 1868 to 1873, and president from 1873 to 1876. This "fine portly gentleman" was a strong supporter of the Society's educational and charitable aims, particularly the Benevolent Fund and the Bell Memorial Scholarships. His *carte-de-visite* (pl. 20) lends support to his reputation as a kind and humorous man.

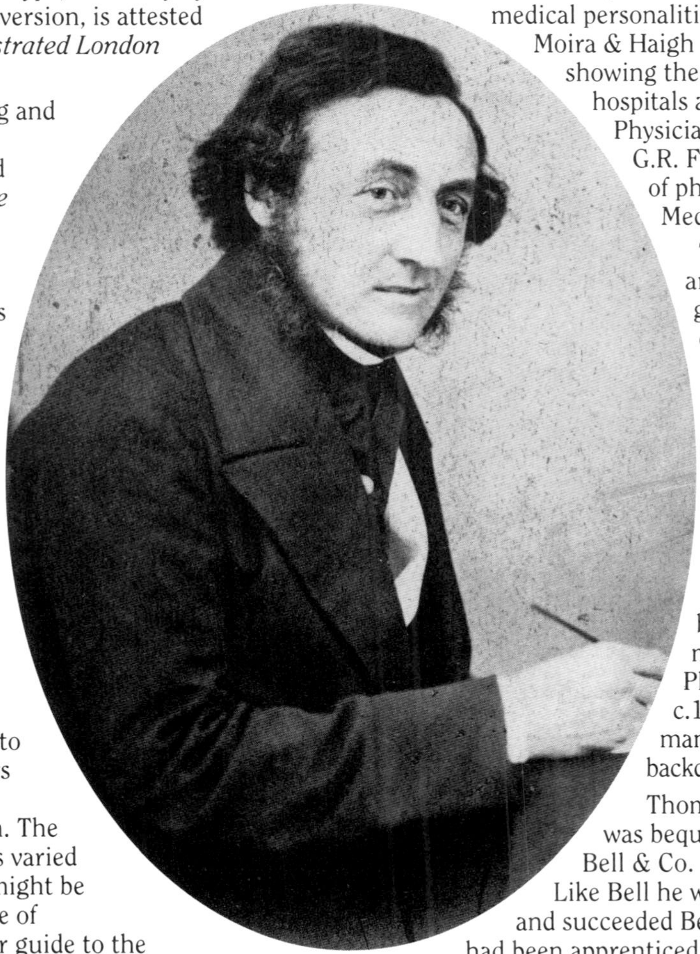

Plate 18.
Jacob Bell as editor of *The Pharmaceutical Journal,* mid 1840s.

11. *The Lancet* 1864 II 283.
12. *The Lancet* 1864 II 621.

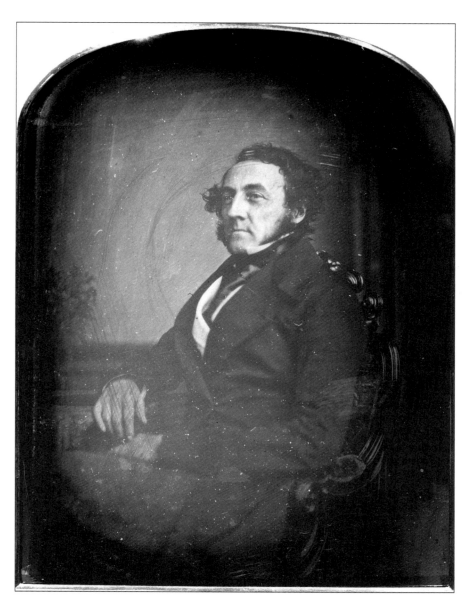

Plate 19.
Jacob Bell, founder of the Pharmaceutical Society of Great Britain, c. 1852.

Regarding Jacob Bell (1810-1859), W.F. Bird said of his evening parties: "The company that he gathered was of a promiscuous character. Bohemia itself, indeed - artists, literary men, actors, actresses in great number, doctors, chemists..."

George Webb Sandford (1813-1892), served his apprenticeship with a Mr Sadler of North Walsham, Norfolk. In 1832 Sandford moved to London and was reluctantly taken on by Alexander Blake for six months, and stayed for 60 years. He joined the Society in 1842 as an Associate, and quickly "attracted the attention of Jacob Bell". The amiable and generous Sandford became a member of Council in 1857, which he remained for 24 years. Elected vice-president in 1861, and then president in 1863, his work in negotiating the passage of the crucial Pharmacy Act of 1868 was acknowledged with a testimonial by subscription in the form of a portrait and silver plate to the value of 500 guineas. T.N.R. Morson, however, mischievously and with some prescience, sent him "a beautiful toy white elephant"

wrapped in a paper inscribed: "Pharmacy act, 1868, by G. W. Sandford. What will he do with it?"

William Lionel Bird (1806-1891), came to London in 1823 to be an apprentice to Mr Pyman, apothecary of Castle Street, to whose business he eventually succeeded. A founder member, he joined the Council in 1848. He was vice-president of the Society for three years though he resigned from the Council in 1867 on being, as he felt, passed over for treasurer.

George Meggeson (1784-1874), a Yorkshireman originally apprenticed in York, came to London to manage the business of Widow Staveley & Co., drug merchants, at 39 Fenchurch Street. He left in 1814 to form the partnership of Cooke, Farley & Meggeson, chemists and druggists, at 61 Cannon Street, which later became Meggeson & Co. Ltd., wholesalers famous for the medicated lozenge "Meggezones". Meggeson joined the Society in 1842, and, on his retirement from business, served on its Council until 1864.

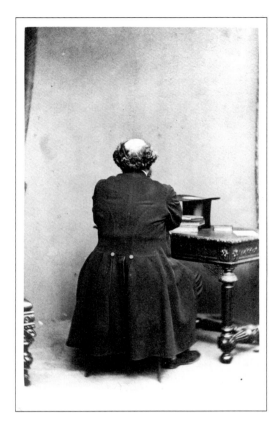

Plate 20.
Thomas Hyde Hills, successor to the firm of John Bell & Co.,
in humorous mood, c.1867.

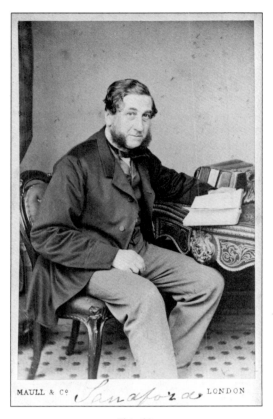

Plate 21.
George Webb Sandford, c.1867

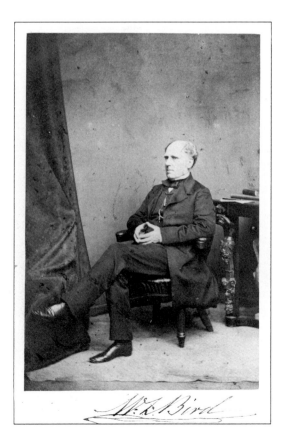

Plate 22.
William L. Bird, c.1867.

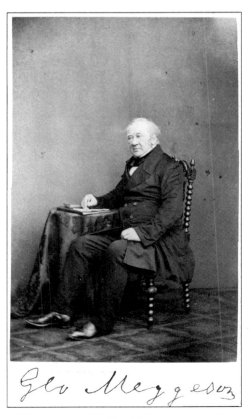

Plate 23.
George Meggeson, c.1864.

George Waugh (1802-1873), vice-president from 1850-51, Waugh several times declined to be president. He was felt to have exercised a restraining influence on his fellow members of Council. However, it was said in his obituary that "He was more given to pass judgement on the measures of others than to originate any himself". Waugh "was one of those well-known London chemists whose names appeared from year to year on the list of its Council, and who were at last thought to partake too much of the character of hereditary councillors".

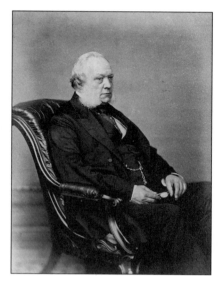

Plate 24.
George Waugh, c. 1865.

Thomas Standring (1802-1874), was apprenticed to Halkyard, an apothecary of Piccadilly, Manchester, to whose business he succeeded, and which he then moved to 1 Piccadilly around 1832. A member of Council from 1847 to 1849, 1858 to 1860, and 1862 to 1869, he was also a visiting apothecary to the Royal Infirmary, and active in Manchester's chemist and druggist associations.

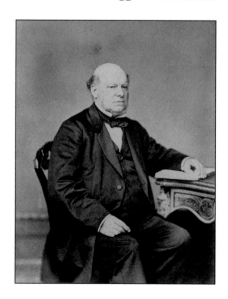

Plate 25.
Thomas Standring, c. 1865.

Henry Deane (1807-1874). A Quaker until his marriage in 1843, he was apprenticed to Joseph Fardon, a chemist and druggist of Reading who had been apprenticed to Deane's uncle before working at John Bell & Co. To the latter pharmacy Deane then progressed, where he stayed for five years, becoming a friend of Jacob and Frederick Bell. During this time he recalled: "we more than once suggested the formation of a society adapted not only for mutual improvement, but with a view to the general improvement of the whole body of chemists and druggists". In 1837 Deane took over a pharmacy at 17 The Pavement, Clapham, a risky venture but with his stoic outlook (he "knew how to live on bread and cheese with no stronger drink than a cup of tea or glass of water"), and his friends' capital, he succeeded. Deane was the first president of the British Pharmaceutical Conference, where his ancient hat, "tall spare form, the gentle countenance and the immemorial costume" were a landmark at these events (pl. 73). He was appointed an examiner in 1844, and elected to Council in 1851; vice-president from 1851-3, and president for 1853-4.

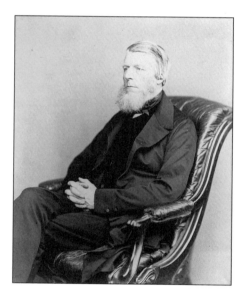

Plate 26.
Henry Deane, c. 1865.

Peter Squire (1798-1884), a major figure in the Pharmaceutical Society, the chemist and druggist to Queen Victoria and the first pharmacist to be on the Royal establishment, is represented in the collection by three portrait photographs, all by noted photographers. These are two *cartes* by Mayall and the famous French portraitist Nadar (pl. 27), and one full-plate print by Maull (pl. 28). Henry Deane spoke highly of Squire's "practical energy" as an examiner, an energy not necessarily appreciated by the students, while it was remarked in his obituaries that "some of his characteristics were too marked to allow him always to escape criticism".

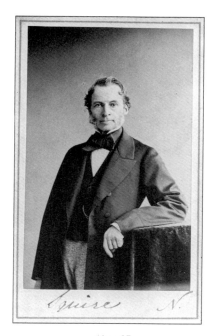

Plate 27.
Peter Squire, c.1860.

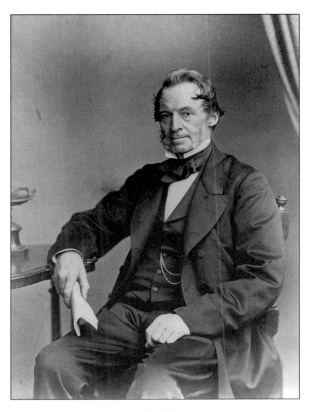

Plate 28.
Peter Squire, c.1865.

Thomas Newborn Robert (T.N.R.) Morson (1799-1874) was apprenticed to a retired army-surgeon in Fleet Market, London, to whose business he succeeded following several years' work in Paris. He became a prominent chemical manufacturer, and the first large-scale British manufacturer of sulphate of quinine and morphia. Morson spent no less than 28 years on the Society's Council, for six of which he was President.

Augustus Bird (d.1900) joined the Society in 1850 following study at the Society's School of Pharmacy. He was an examiner from 1853 to 1872 when he was replaced by William Martindale (pl. 32). Bird's pharmacy was at 22 Kensington High Street.

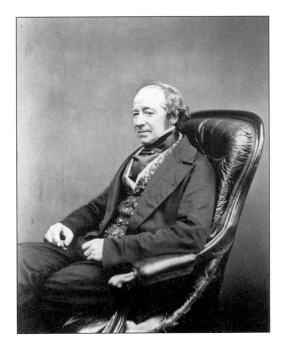

Plate 29.
Thomas N.R. Morson, c.1865.

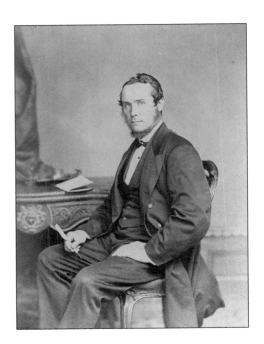

Plate 30.
Augustus Bird, c.1865.

Theophilus Redwood (1806-1892) came to John Bell & Co. in 1823 following his Cardiff apprenticeship. There he became "the inseparable companion" of Jacob Bell. On the establishment of the Pharmaceutical Society's School in 1842, Redwood was appointed the first Professor of Pharmacy. He designed the 1845 basement laboratory at 17 Bloomsbury Square, the first of its type in Britain devoted to pharmacy, as well as the later laboratory on the top floor. Redwood wrote many works on pharmacy, edited the *British Pharmacopoeia*, and was sub-editor of Bell's *Pharmaceutical Journal*. He married the eldest daughter of T.N.R. Morson.

William Martindale (1840-1902) studied at the School of Pharmacy after serving his apprenticeship in his native Carlisle. He became an assistant at Morson and Son, then dispenser and teacher of pharmacy at University College Hospital and demonstrator of materia medica at University College. In 1873 he started his business in New Cavendish Street. An examiner from 1873 to 1882, he became a member of Council in 1889, treasurer of the Society in 1898, and president in 1899. The first edition of his now famous *Extra Pharmacopoeia* was published in 1883.

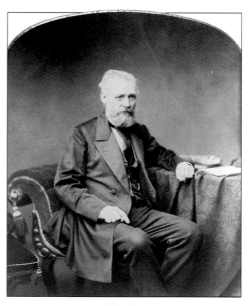

Plate 31.
Professor Theophilus Redwood, c.1870.

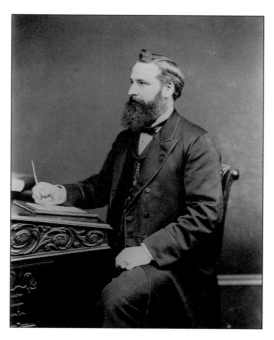

Plate 32.
William Martindale, 1879.

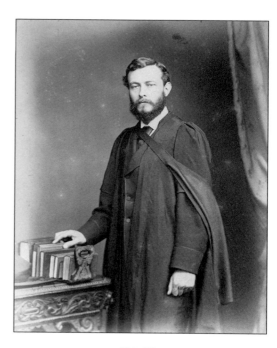

Plate 33.
Dr William A. Tilden, 1872.

Sir William Augustus Tilden (1842-1926) attended the Society's School and the Royal College of Chemistry. He was the first Bell Scholar, becoming a junior assistant at Stenhouse's private laboratory and then a demonstrator at the Society's School from 1863 to 1872. Later a senior science master at Clifton College, Tilden eventually became Professor of Chemistry at Mason College, Birmingham and at the Royal College of Chemistry. Of his time as a Bell Scholar he later remarked, "I owe nothing whatever in the way of teaching to the scholarship, except the money, for during the session the Professor [Redwood] appeared only twice. The first time he came to receive the fees.... The second time he was showing some stranger round the place...."

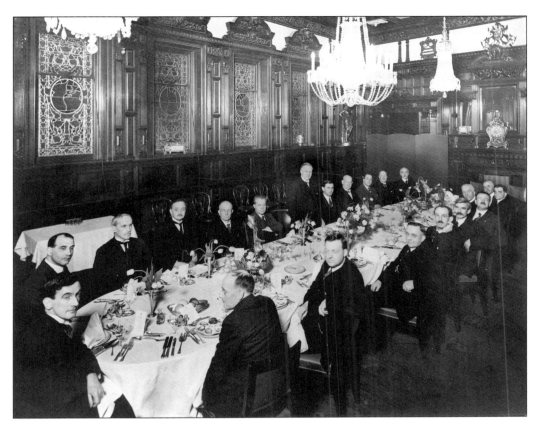

Plate 34.
A Pharmaceutical Society Council dinner at the Holborn Restaurant, 1925/1926.

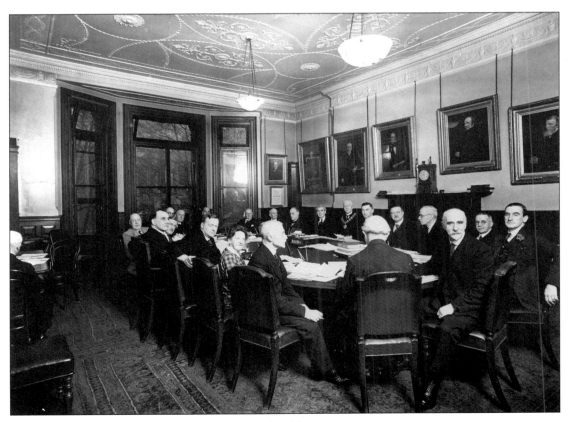

Plate 35.
Meeting of the 1931/1932 Council of the Pharmaceutical Society at 17 Bloomsbury Square, London.

18

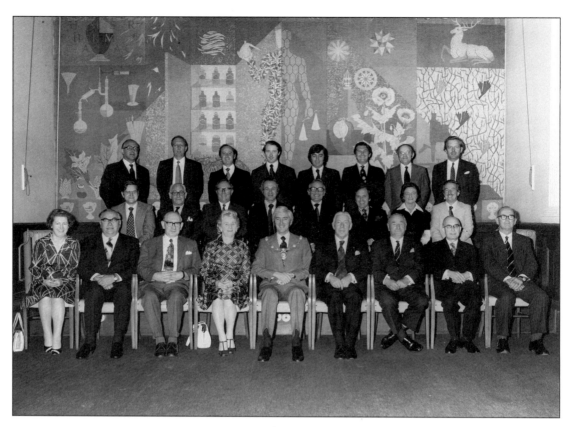

Plate 36.
Council of the Pharmaceutical Society, 17 Bloomsbury Square, London, 1975.

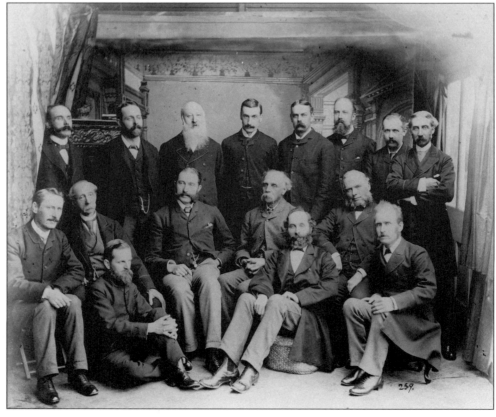

Plate 37.
The Bristol Pharmaceutical Association, c.1890.

# JACOB BELL MEMORIAL SCHOLARS

In July 1861 the Council of the Society adopted the arrangements put forward for the Jacob Bell Memorial Scholarships. The original proposal to establish this award in 1859 led to an appeal that raised £2,000, enabling the Council to offer two scholarships of £30 on an annual basis.

Portraits of recipients of the award between 1861 and 1970 are assembled in an album of photographs held by the Society, the early scholars recorded in *carte-de-visite* and later as photographic postcards. These youthful portraits include many future pharmacists who became distinguished members of their profession.

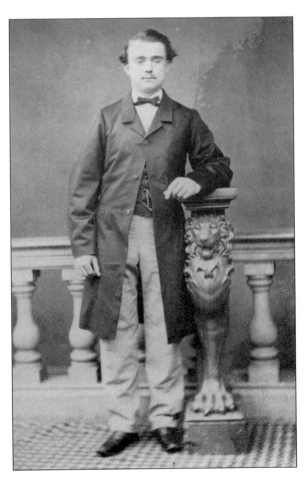

Plate 38.
Jacob Bell memorial scholar, Charles Umney, 1862.

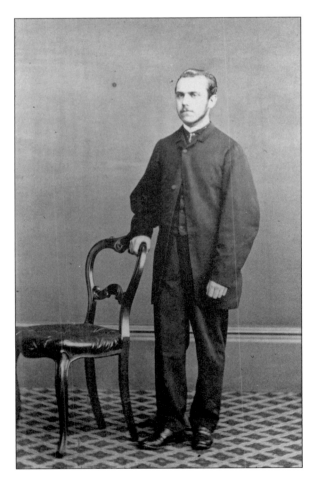

Plate 39.
Jacob Bell memorial scholar, Alfred Neobard Palmer, 1867.

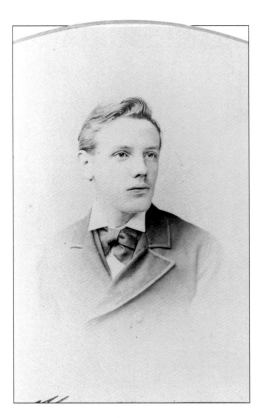

Plate 40.
Jacob Bell memorial scholar, Henry George Greenish, 1875.

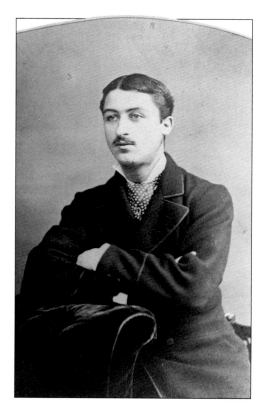

Plate 41.
Jacob Bell memorial scholar, John Leaver West, 1875.

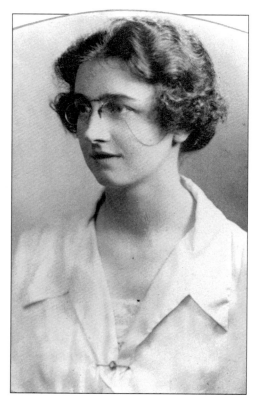

Plate 42.
Jacob Bell memorial scholar, Joyce M. Carr, 1921.

# BENEVOLENT FUND

The formation of a benevolent fund ("to provide ... for the relief of the distressed members and associates of the Society and of their Widows and Orphans") was among the original objects of the Pharmaceutical Society's Charter. Since 1865 the fund has supplied annuitants with a fixed income and has also made individual grants to those in need.

The collection of photographic portraits of annuitants provides a remarkable social record: the stock pose of these *carte-de-visite* and postcard images often betrays little of the applicants' reduced financial and social circumstances in contrast with the known details of hardship that befell some of these chemists and druggists and their dependents. Many of the portraits seem to have been taken several years before the subjects made their application to the fund (pl. 43 and 45).

It appears that little effort was made to respect the confidentiality of those who applied to the fund during the nineteenth century, as elections to select worthy annuitants were open to all members and associates of the Society and to contributors to the fund.

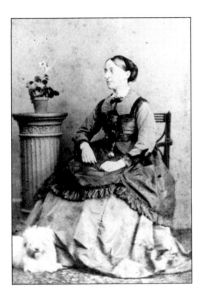

Plate 43.
Harriett M. Bensley, annuitant of Pharmaceutical Society Benevolent Fund in 1891, taken c.1860.

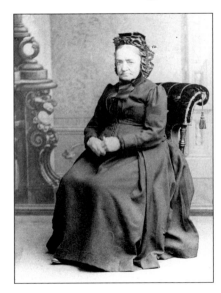

Plate 44.
R. Mowbray, annuitant of Pharmaceutical Society
Benevolent Fund in 1891, c.1891.

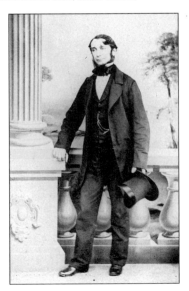

Plate 45.
G. Foster, annuitant of Pharmaceutical Society
Benevolent Fund in 1897, c.1860.

# PHARMACY EDUCATION AND SCHOOLS OF PHARMACY

The establishment of the School of Pharmacy in 1842 was among the earliest and most significant acts of the Society's founders. From it evolved the basis of systematic training for pharmacy as a scientific profession, ultimately replacing apprenticeship by degree courses undertaken by all qualified pharmacists today.

Committed to "promoting a uniform system of education" for pharmacy, the Council of the Society envisaged the School as a model for the preparation of students as qualified practitioners and a centre for pharmaceutical research. It became a School of the University of London in 1925, though the majority of the finance continued to be provided by the Society until after the 1939-1945 war. In 1949 the University purchased from the Society the new Brunswick Square building built for the Society (pl. 64) and assumed responsibility for its funding. The first lectures, started in February 1842, were offered in medical botany, chemistry, materia medica and pharmacy, while in 1844 the Society's School became the first in Britain to offer practical instruction in chemistry under the direction of Professor Theophilus Redwood. But in spite of the early advances in pharmacy education and research pioneered in Bloomsbury, the establishment of similar schools outside London was slow. Only with the Pharmacy Act of 1868 (which brought enforced qualification by examination for those wishing to register as a chemist and druggist or pharmaceutical chemist) did the number of private, and later institutional schools, in London and the provinces, grow appreciably.

The earliest views are notable for their detailed record of the chemical laboratory opened on the third floor of 17 Bloomsbury Square in 1861 (pl. 48-50). Among the students at work in their appointed places are the two Bell Scholars of 1883/4, F. McDiarmid and R. W. Pierce. Meanwhile, the original basement laboratory was converted into a store and the School lecture theatre, which it remained until 1957. The horseshoe form of the lecturer's bench was modelled on that used by Michael Faraday at the Royal Institution (pl. 57).

The Society's School is the subject of a substantial group of photographs, covering over a century of its history,

including a personal collection formed by Dr T.E. Wallis, lecturer in botany, and later reader in pharmacognosy and curator of the Society's museum (pl. 53). Formal and informal shots illustrate the changing appearance of the School. They record the varied life of the pharmacy student in the context of the laboratory and lecture theatre set against a backdrop of Bloomsbury Square. Staff, too, of all ranks and grades share a place among the images that depict the School and its activities.

Private or proprietary schools provided a variety of courses on a full and part-time basis leading to the minor and major qualifying examinations. Of these, the London College of Pharmacy was one of the best known. It had been founded in 1899 by Henry Wootton and earned one of the best examination records of any school.

Scriven J. Turner (d. 1986), who was among one of the last generations of students to study at the College before its closure as the last private school in London in 1945, compiled a scrapbook of his student days. An informal shot records a group of his contemporaries reading the latest edition of the *Argus,* a well read College newspaper (pl.66). It first appeared in 1928 as a single weekly sheet and became, by 1933, a 16 page weekly magazine with a circulation rising to 500 by 1939.

In 1918 the principle of a compulsory course of study was introduced. Previously there had been no control of the curriculum taught by the schools of pharmacy or the length of time required for a student to study in preparation for their examinations. At this time it also became necessary for schools that were to train ex-service students in receipt of a government grant to be recognised by the Society. In combination, these measures led to raised standards in the modern technical education provided by the institutional schools, and the demise of the private or proprietary schools.

Since 1967, it has been required that to register as a pharmacist, it is necessary to hold a pharmacy degree approved by the Society and to complete a satisfactory period of pre-registration experience.

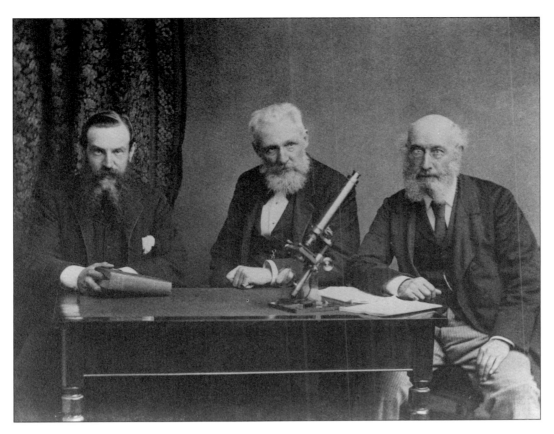

Plate 46.
"The Last Watch of Hero": Professors Attfield, Redwood, and Bentley, c.1881-1887.

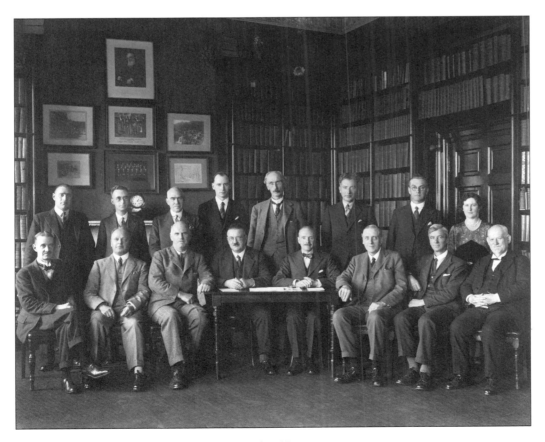

Plate 47.
Pharmaceutical Society board of examiners for Scotland, Scottish Branch, York Place, Edinburgh, 1933.

24

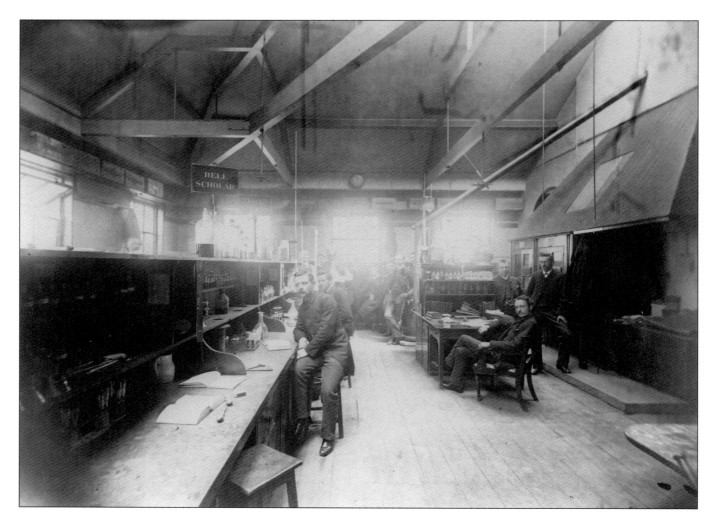

Plate 48.
Chemical laboratory, third floor, 17 Bloomsbury Square, 1883/4.

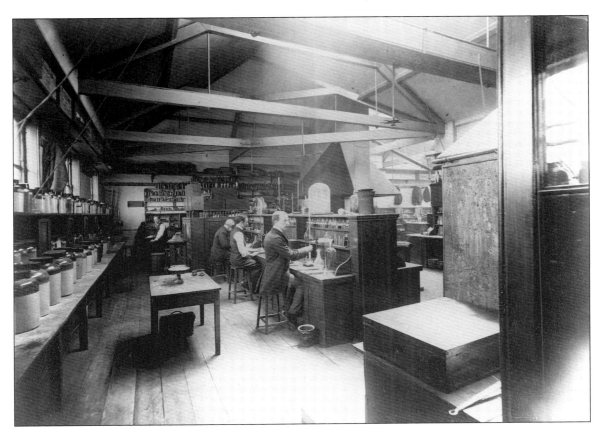

Plate 49.
The "major chemical laboratory", third floor, 17 Bloomsbury Square, 1883/4.

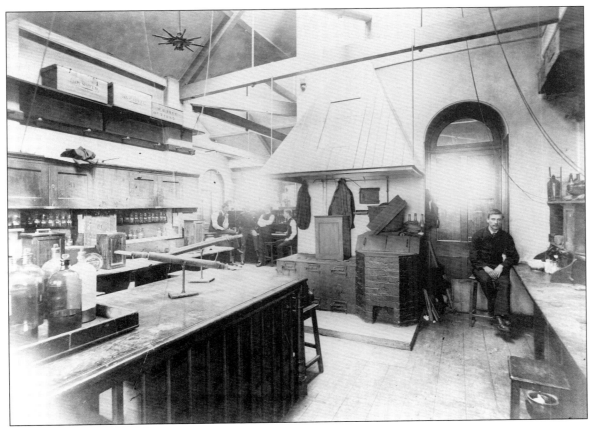

Plate 50.
The laboratory steward's bench in the major chemical laboratory, third floor,
17 Bloomsbury Square, 1883/4.

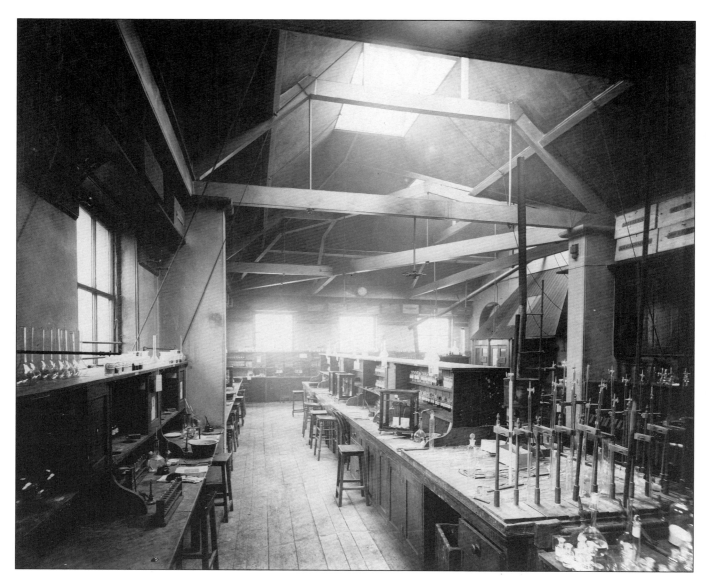

Plate 51.
The "chemical laboratory", third floor, 17 Bloomsbury Square, 1892.

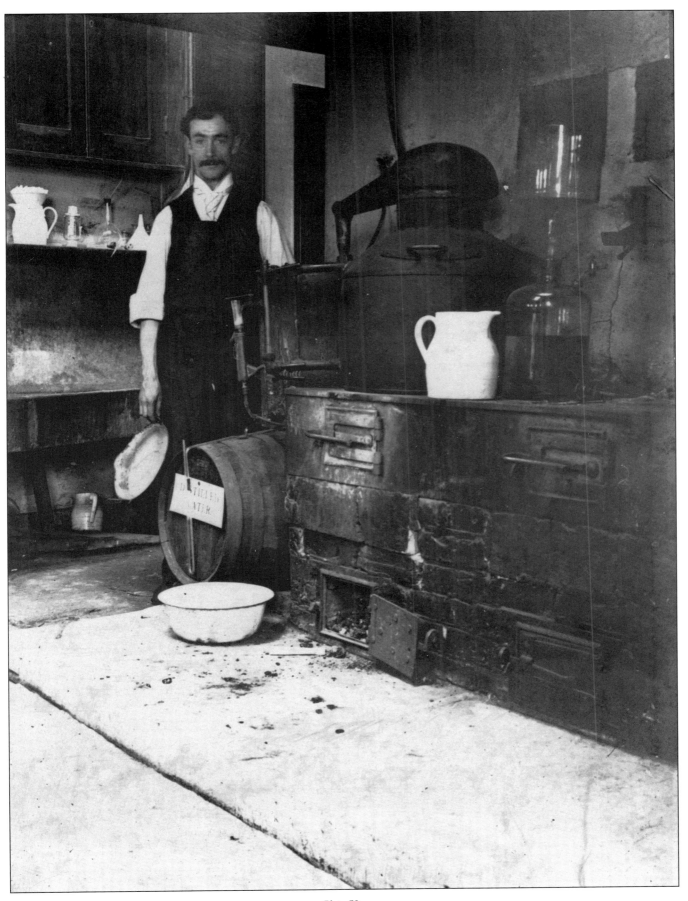

Plate 52.
The old still in the chemistry laboratory with the laboratory assistant H. Caines,
17 Bloomsbury Square, c. 1901.

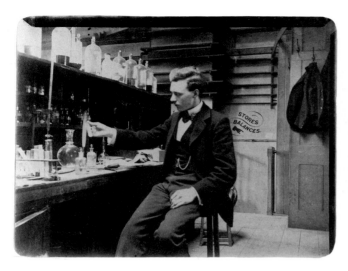

Plate 53.
Dr T.E. Wallis in the chemistry laboratory at
17 Bloomsbury Square, 1898.

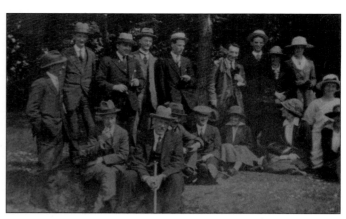

Plate 54.
A botanical ramble by the School on Hayes Common
led by Professor H.G. Greenish, 1921.

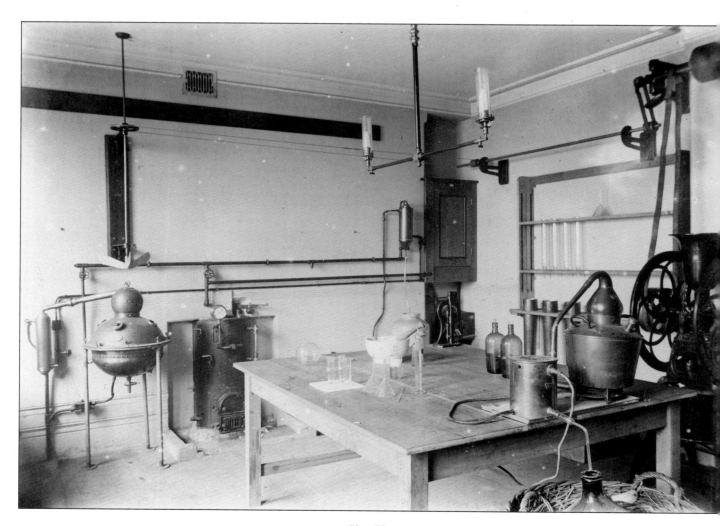

Plate 55.
"Laboratory for applied pharmaceutics showing layout with two copper stills, steam heated pan etc.",
17 Bloomsbury Square, c.1901-1904.

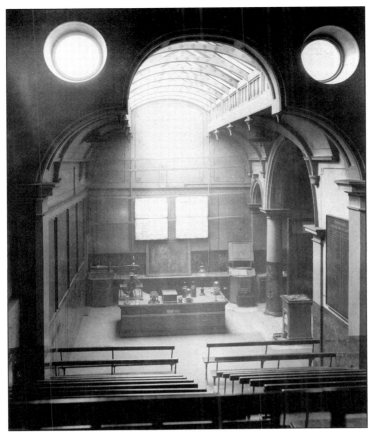

Plate 56.
The lecture theatre of the School of Pharmacy, 17 Bloomsbury Square, 1892.

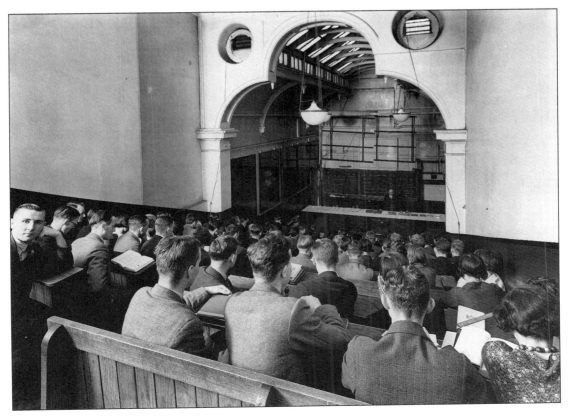

Plate 57.
The lecture theatre of the School of Pharmacy with Professor Greenish lecturing, 1931.

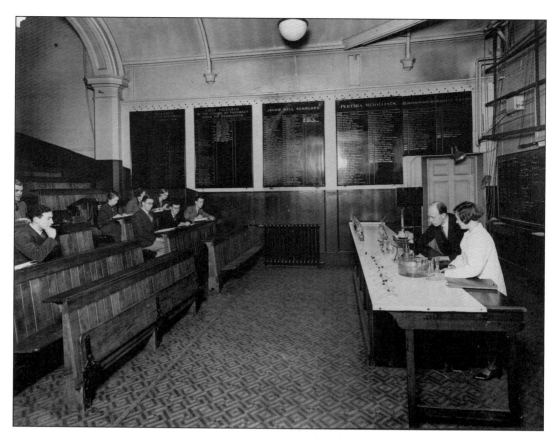

Plate 58.
The modernised lecture theatre at the School of Pharmacy, with W.H. Linnell speaking, c.1931.

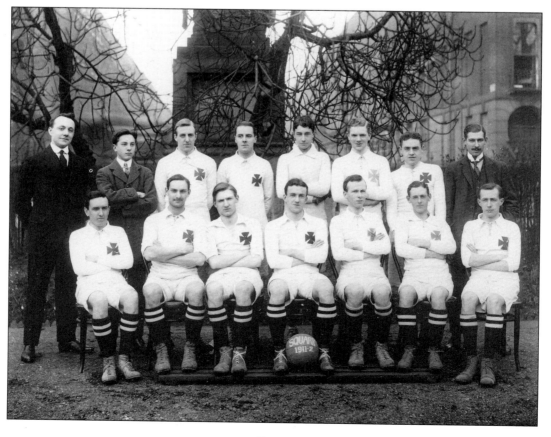

Plate 59.
Group photograph of the School of Pharmacy football team, Bloomsbury Square, 1911/1912.

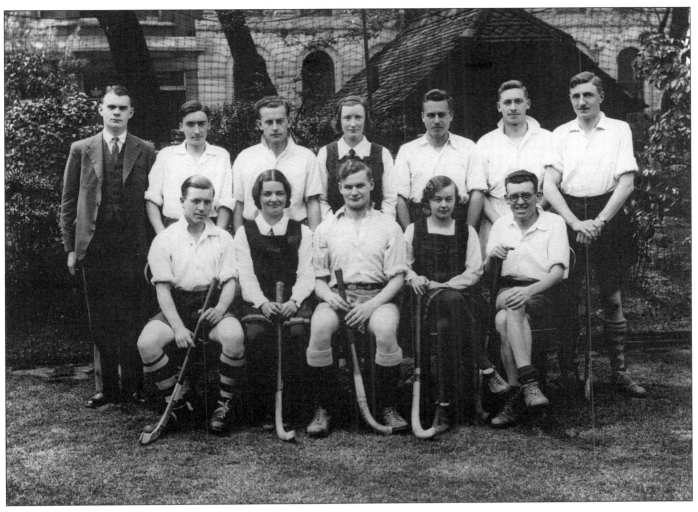

Plate 60.
Group photograph of the School of Pharmacy hockey team, Bloomsbury Square, 1934/1935.

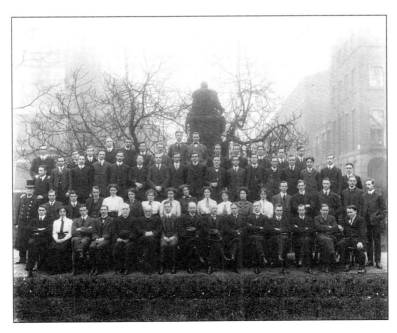

Plate 61.
Group photograph of students and staff of the School of Pharmacy, 17 Bloomsbury Square, London, c.1907.

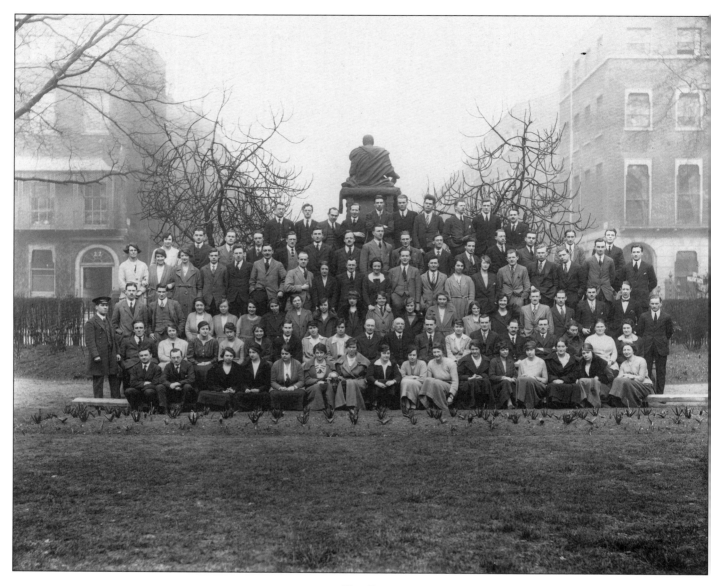

Plate 62.
Group photograph of students and staff of the School of Pharmacy, 1921/1922.

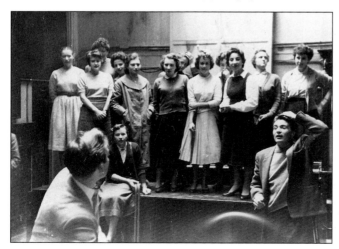

Plate 63.
The students peculiar ritual leg-examination at the School of Pharmacy,
17 Bloomsbury Square, 1963/1964.

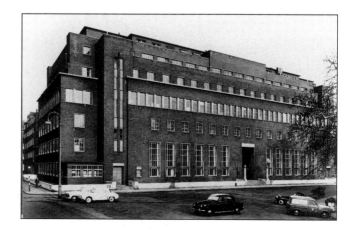

Plate 64.
The School of Pharmacy at Brunswick Square, originally intended to be
the new headquarters of the Pharmaceutical Society, 1950s.

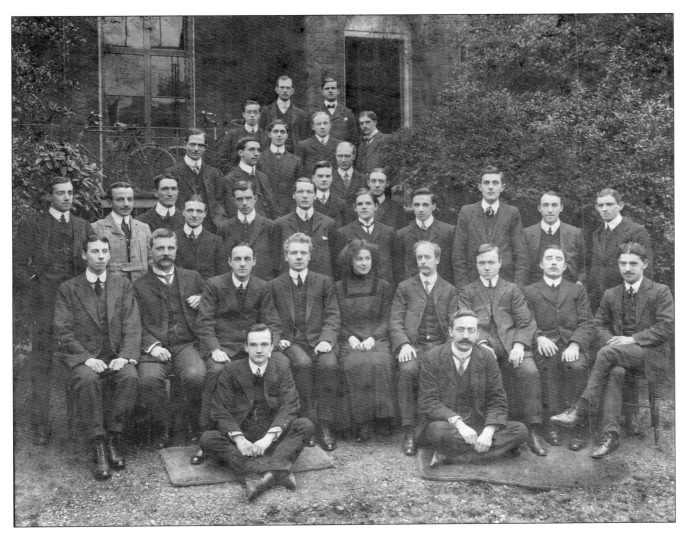

Plate 65.
School group, the Metropolitan College of Pharmacy, 160/162 Kennington Park Road, London, c.1905.

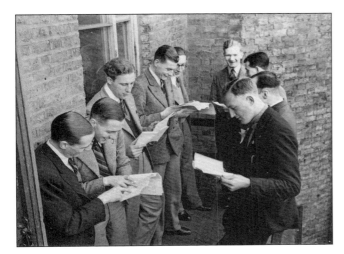

Plate 66.
*Argus* day, at the South London School of Pharmacy, 1940.

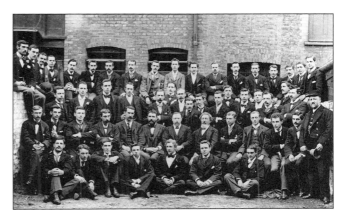

Plate 67.
Group photograph of Muter's College (South London School of Pharmacy),
London, 1896.

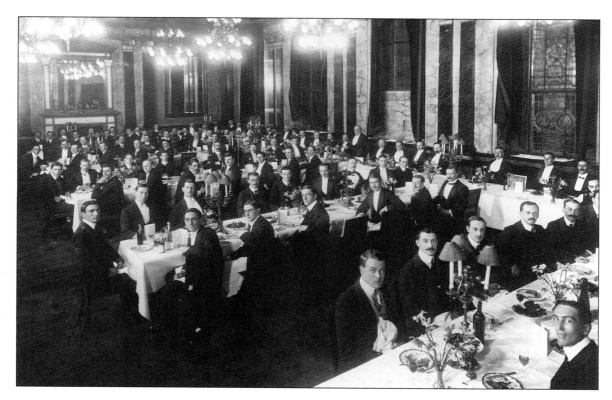

Plate 68.
The annual dinner of the South of England College of Pharmacy, The Holborn Restaurant, London, 9 June 1910.

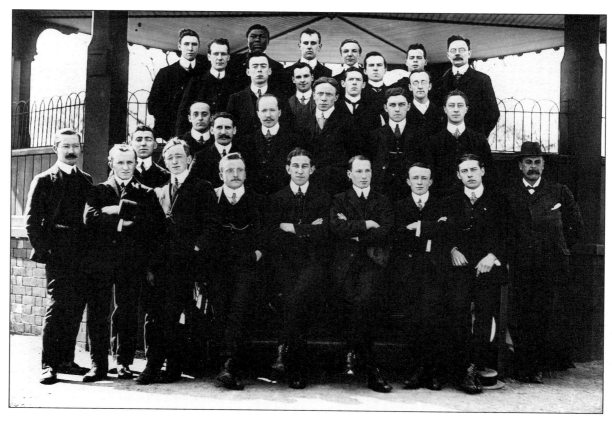

Plate 69.
Students of the Manchester School of Pharmacy, c. 1900.

# CONFERENCES AND MEETINGS

Formal and informal group photographs to mark meetings, conferences and congresses of all kinds are well represented within the Society's collection. From the beginning the Society's founders were eager to cultivate relations with their foreign counterparts, both through personal contacts of members and with national and international organisations representing the interests of pharmacy.

## INTERNATIONAL

The first International Pharmaceutical Congress was held in 1864. Seventeen years later the Pharmaceutical Society was host to the Fifth International Pharmacy Congress in London where subjects under discussion included proposals for an International Pharmacopoeia. About 150 of those attending took part in "a most agreeable excursion from London to Henley-on-Thames and thence by water to Maidenhead" (pl. 70). An album of *cartes,* which is part of the Society's collection, showing 102 of the participants was assembled to commemorate the Congress.

In May 1929, the Fifth International Congress of Military Medicine and Pharmacy was held in London. This gathering was attended by 750 delegates from 40 nations and the pharmaceutical section, mainly comprising pharmaceutical officers of foreign armies, met in the lecture theatre of 17 Bloomsbury Square (pl. 71). The "horizon blue and field grey uniforms gave a note of unwonted colour to Bloomsbury Square" in this "most striking group".

The International Pharmaceutical Federation met in Paris in 1953 where Sir Hugh Linstead, secretary and registrar of the Pharmaceutical Society, was appointed president of the Federation for the forthcoming meeting of 1955 in London (pl. 72).

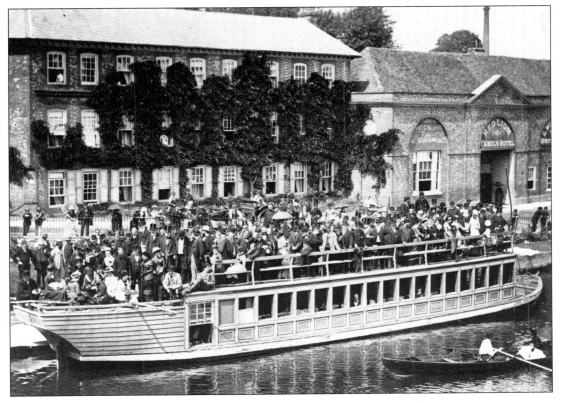

Plate 70.
Riverboat excursion,
Henley-on-Thames International Pharmacy Congress, London, 1881.

36

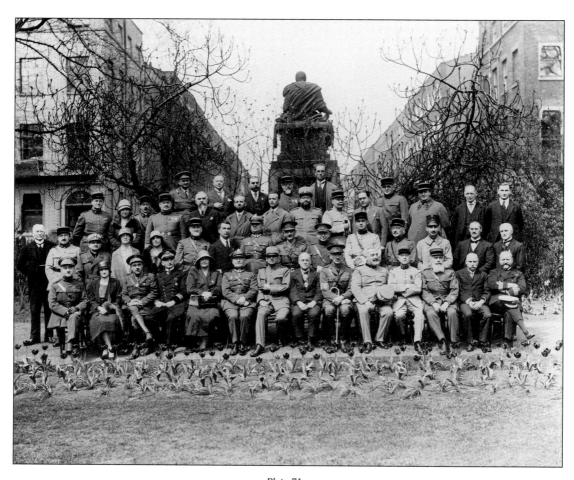

Plate 71.
Delegates to the Fifth International Congress of Military Medicine,
seated in Bloomsbury Square, London, 10 May, 1929.

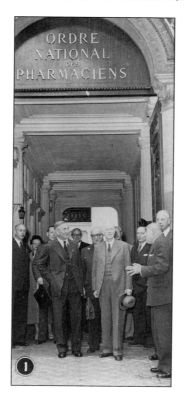

Plate 72.
Members of the Bureau, including Sir Hugh Linstead, Dr E. Höst (president), and Dr H. Birza (general secretary)
at the Ordre National des Pharmaciens International Pharmaceutical Federation, Paris, 1953.

# BRITISH PHARMACEUTICAL CONFERENCE

Some of the most engaging images that record the British Pharmaceutical Conference (or BPC as it is commonly known) depict the social activities and excursions organised for delegates and their companions: formal groups as well as snapshots illustrate the "friendly reunion" (an original object of the Conference) that became an established feature of the meetings.

The idea of a regular scientific meeting for chemists and druggists was first raised in 1852 by G.F. Schact of Bristol but it took 11 years before the initial gathering of the British Pharmaceutical Conference was held in Newcastle. The inaugural session took place during the meeting of the British Association in September 1863. Like the American Pharmaceutical Association and the British Association, the object of the British Pharmaceutical Conference was to hold a regular meeting in different provincial cities at which subjects of mutual pharmaceutical interest would be considered. A separate organisation from the Society was founded to convene and arrange this conference on an annual basis. Its membership was not to be confined exclusively to members of the Pharmaceutical Society even though it was made plain from the start that an object of the BPC would be "to promote the interests of the Society". Only in 1923 was an agreement reached that the BPC, under the Society's auspices would be controlled by an independent Committee, elected by members of the Conference with the Society represented by its president and three members of Council. The Society assumed responsibility to publish the *Yearbook of Pharmacy* (in which the transactions were published) which became the *Journal of Pharmacy and Pharmacology* in 1949. Since 1970 the organisation of the Conference has been undertaken by the Organisation Committee of Council, through which the Conference Science Committee and the Local Organising Committee report to Council.

One of the most striking conference groups was taken against the backdrop of Tintern Abbey when 250 took part in an all-day excursion organised for the Bristol BPC of 1903 (pl.74). *The Pharmaceutical Journal* reports that tea was served in a "capacious tent" and "a few songs were given towards the end of tea, Mr E. W. Hills presiding at the piano... The photographic group... is being sold by Mr Boorne, the Hon. Secretary of the Local Committee at the following prices: un-mounted 3s 6d (postage 3d extra); mounted, 4s 6d (postage 6d extra)."

Increasingly elaborate arrangements were made for delegates and their companions to benefit from their stay in the location of the conference. The social events and outings held for the 38th annual meeting in Dublin in 1901 included opportunities to take part in a *conversazione* at the Science and Arts Museum, a drive on the electric trams, a drawing room concert, a smoking concert, a visit to the Botanic Gardens, luncheon in the Mansion House and an excursion to the Guinness factory. It was usual for a variety of recreational events to be arranged for wives accompanying delegates, often organised by a ladies' committee. According to the Conference programme for 1901 "...we can safely predict that the fair visitors will have charming recollections of Dublin" (pl.76).

Another evocative photograph was taken at the Old Mill Jesmond Dene, Newcastle-upon-Tyne, 1909, where delegates and their companions posed, "ranged among the rocks and waterfalls" (pl.75).

Many of the surviving pictures of the early conferences were taken by local photographers, sometimes pharmacists who specialised in photography. The snapshot of a conference visit to the Roman Baths, Bath in 1924 is probably one of a series taken by Mr John Cleworth, a "photographic chemist" of Manchester whose photographs from various conferences were reproduced in the pharmaceutical press over a number of years. John Cleworth had been apprenticed in Manchester and studied at the Northern College of Pharmacy and "Duncan's" in Edinburgh. In 1901 he had purchased a failing branch pharmacy at 56 Ducie Street, Manchester. Cleworth's concentration on the photographic side of his business (and through specialising in "own-name" photographic chemicals), had by 1907 turned the pharmacy into "the smartest and most interesting in Manchester". His daily displays of new photographs of local interest were a popular attraction for passing commuters, and photographic postcards of the day's events could be purchased the same evening.

The tradition of capturing moments of recreation at BPCs is still a feature of the press photography at this annual event. Reproduced in the pages of *The Pharmaceutical Journal* and *The Chemist and Druggist* to enliven the reporting of conference proceedings, the images of often familiar personalities add a sometimes humorous and personal dimension to the conference records.

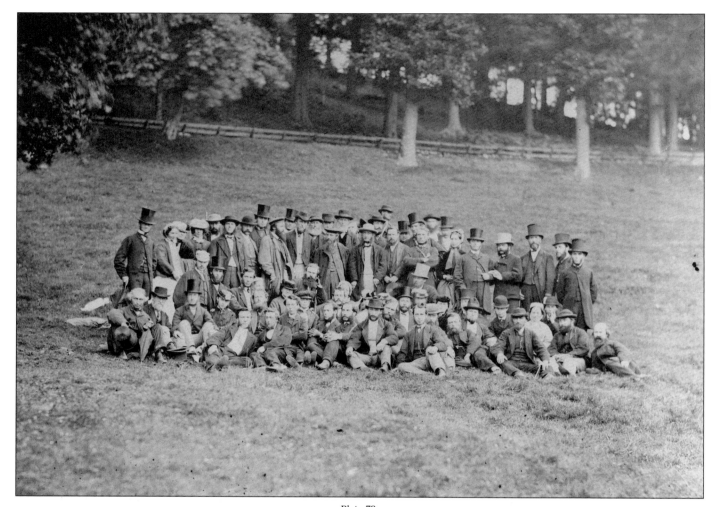

Plate 73.
The British Pharmaceutical Conference, Dundee, visit to Craighall, Blairgowrie, Perth,
5 September 1867.

Conference reports in the pharmaceutical press supply
details of the events at which some of these photographs
were taken: the earliest BPC photograph in the collection
recalls a picnic excursion to Craighall at the Dundee
meeting of September 1867. A reporter of *The Dundee
Advertiser,* quoted by *The Pharmaceutical Journal,*
describes how the party, who travelled in a large omnibus
and four wagonettes, enjoyed "a sumptuous dinner supplied
by Miss McGregor of the Temperance Hotel, Blairgowrie".
Afterwards "the greater portion were disposed in a group
with a view to being photographed by Mr Abbott".

39

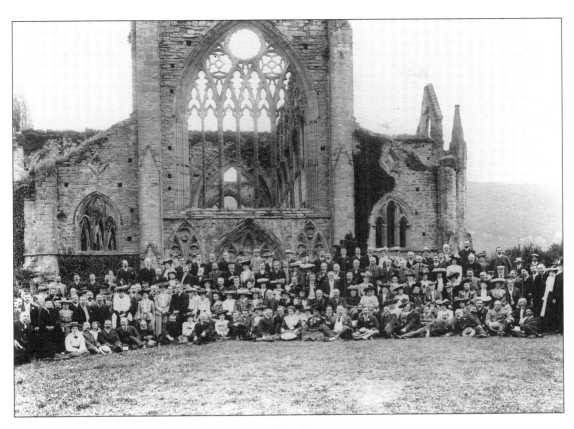

Plate 74.
British Pharmaceutical Conference, Bristol, 1903. The visit to Tintern Abbey, Monmouthshire, 30 July 1903.

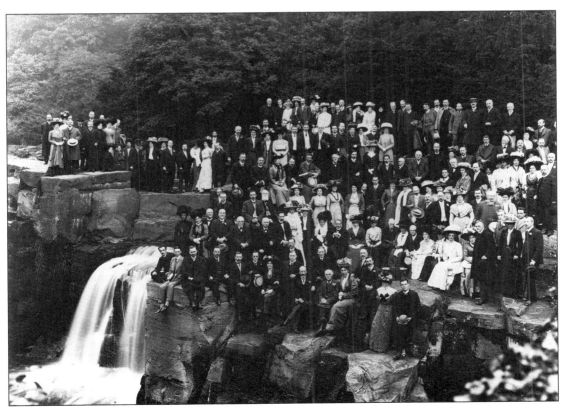

Plate 75.
British Pharmaceutical Conference, Newcastle-upon-Tyne, Group photograph taken at Jesmond Dene, 27 July 1909.

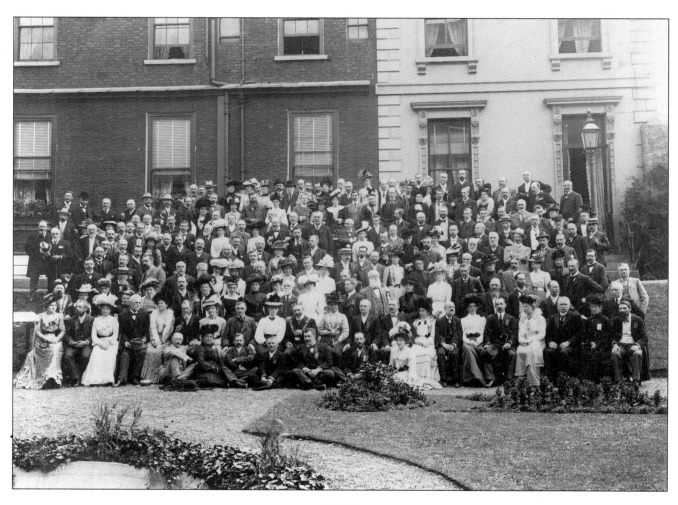

Plate 76.
British Pharmaceutical Conference, Dublin, 31 July 1901.

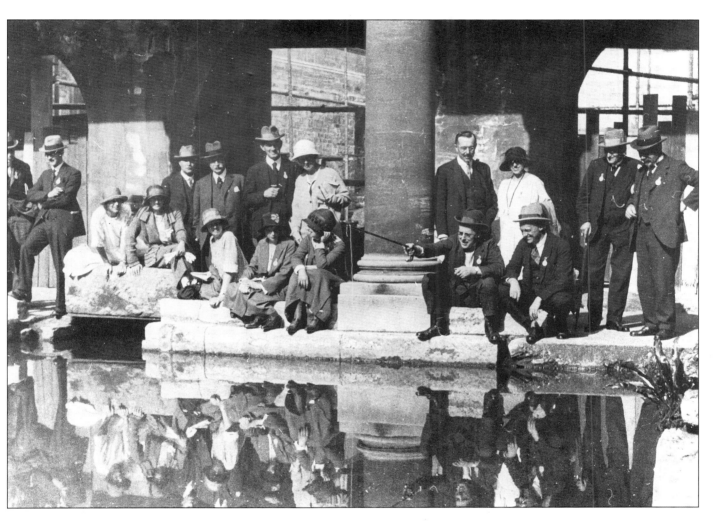

Plate 77.
British Pharmaceutical Conference, Bath. Visit to the Roman Baths, 1924.

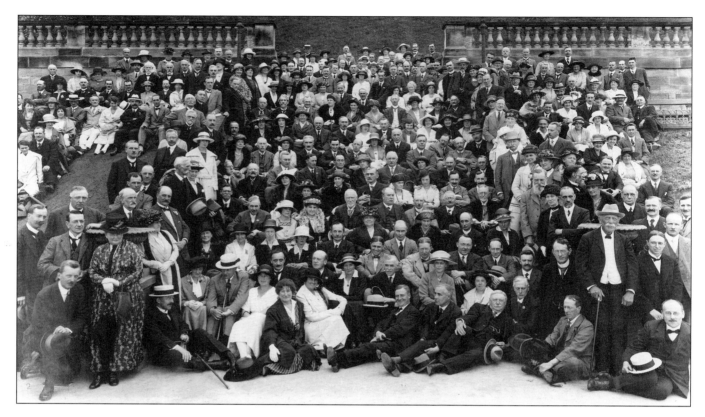

Plate 78.
British Pharmaceutical Conference, Scarborough Spa, Yorkshire, 15 June 1921.

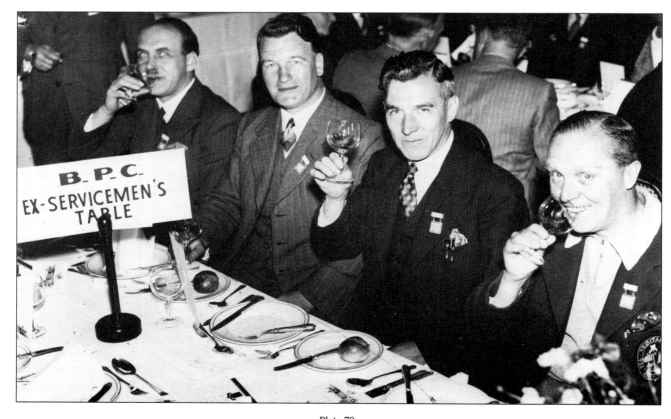

Plate 79.
"At Tuesday's Luncheon", the BPC Ex-Servicemen's Table, British Pharmaceutical Conference, Liverpool, 27 July 1937.

43

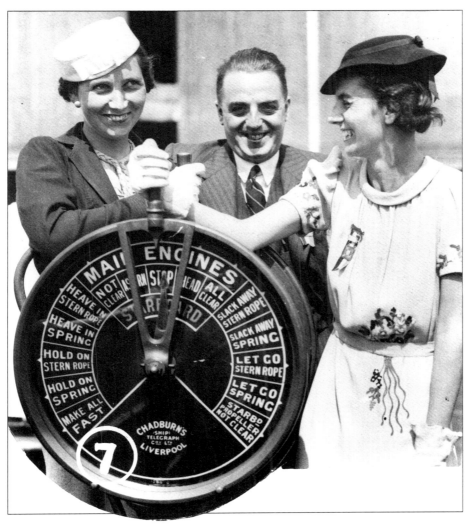

Plate 80.
"Visitors on Board a Liner, Miss Smail with Mr and Mrs Clubb". British Pharmaceutical Conference visit to Birkenhead. 1937.

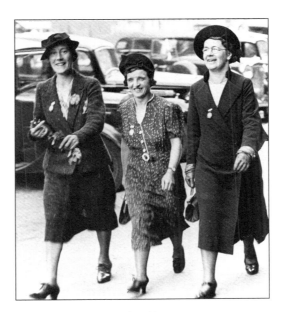

Plate 81.
The Peebles Excursion: "Hurrying for the bus", British Pharmaceutical Conference, Edinburgh, 1938.

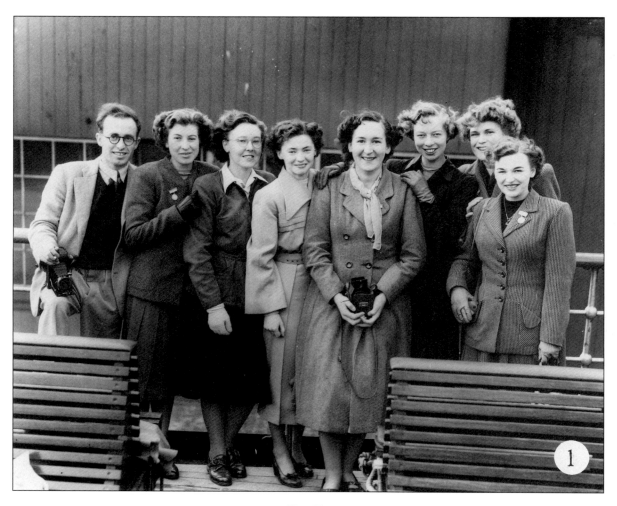

Plate 82.
"The Excursion down the Clyde. A group of young hospital pharmacists".
British Pharmaceutical Conference, Edinburgh, September 1950.

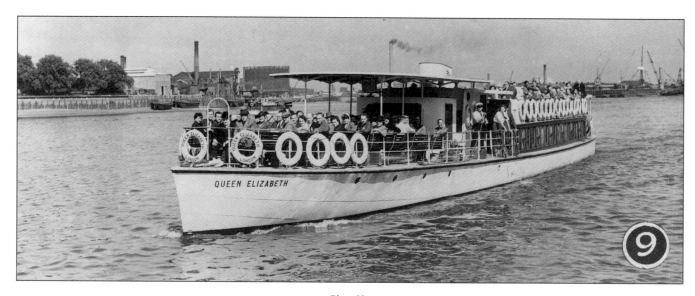

Plate 83.
"The River Excursion from Westminster to Greenwich Pier. The second boat arriving at Greenwich Pier".
British Pharmaceutical Conference, London, 3 September 1953.

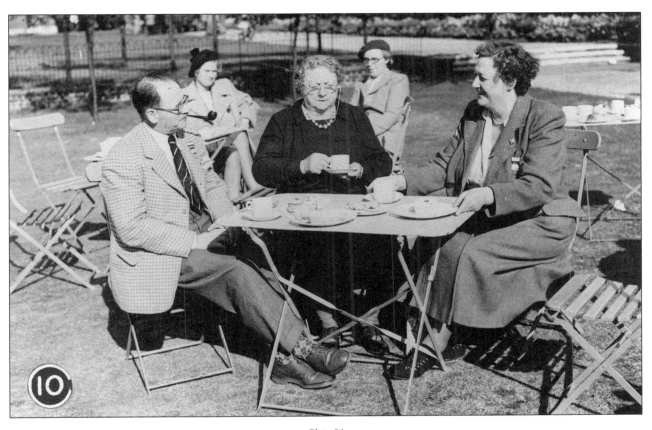

Plate 84.
"The River Excursion from Westminster to Greenwich Pier.
The Chairman of the Conference with his mother and sister".
British Pharmaceutical Conference, London, National Maritime Museum, 2 September 1953.

# PHARMACY PREMISES

In nearly every instance, photographs of pharmacy premises in the Society's collection were taken to commemorate a specific event. Principally this was the opening or refurbishment of a pharmacy, in which case the typical image is of the building's frontage, and the commissioning proprietor will almost always appear standing proudly, if rather awkwardly, on the doorstep (pl. 117). Interior views of this type are less common until later in the twentieth century, presumably because of lighting difficulties. Otherwise, the photographs were intended to record the appearance of an old-fashioned, or "traditional" pharmacy and its fittings, or perhaps to show a picturesque laboratory (pl. 86, 91). The majority of these images therefore were intended to depict the unusual or uncommon; the new, the remarkable, or the antique, and for this reason impromptu photographs of the workaday pharmacy or areas other than the front-shop or laboratory are extremely rare. Photographs of the storerooms, cellars, drying rooms or powdering rooms are almost unknown.

However, the Society's photographic collection reflects the great diversity of pharmacies, whether that of the long-established "historic house", the orthodox proprietor/owner, the multiples and the cash chemists, prosperous or poor. The concept of the appearance of the "traditional" pharmacy, once merely associated with that of the previous generation, has now become firmly identified with that of the late nineteenth or early twentieth century. In some ways this is misleading, since pharmacies have, of course, evolved to meet the changing needs of the profession and of their customers. In doing so they have reflected in their appearance contemporary tastes and fashions in design, layout, and decoration. These changes can be traced in some detail from the photographic collection, though very few images preserve the appearance of the late Georgian shopfront, with its two old-fashioned bay windows, lost to the six-paned plate-glass front in the 1840s.

Theophilus Redwood considered that the dispensary should be "a fit place for healthful recreation, instead of being, as it too often is, an imperfectly-heated and badly ventilated apartment, where body and mind are benumbed with cold or oppressed with vitiated air". The ideal dispensary had to have ample light, though without direct sunlight and so without large windows, and with easy access. Steps of any kind were thought to discourage customers and were often removed.

The limited number of specialist pharmaceutical shopfitters, such as S. Maw, Son & Sons, ensured an almost universal style of design in Britain and the Empire during the late nineteenth century. During this time the "traditional" appearance of the pharmacy was established, and it was often observed that "Many successful businesses owe not a little to the clever way in which the shopfitter has made the interior and exterior of the premises attractive".

In pharmacies of this date there was "the usual tramway" for carboys of coloured water, which were sometimes provided with oil lamps or gas jets to illuminate them at night and cast an attractive multi-coloured glow into the street. There was usually an outside lamp in coloured glass. The exterior, often of mahogany or teak was frequently painted in a solid dark colour, usually black or green with a simple name in gold letters above mosaic-floored entrances, marble steps, and red granite footings. The interior was treated in a similar fashion, with mahogany fittings and sometimes false enamelled iron ceilings decorated with raised patterns.

The album of excellent photographs produced for the firm of Heppell & Co. in 1912 records in extraordinary detail the interior and exterior views of the London branches of this "high-class", modern, metropolitan business. The firm, incorporated in 1924, had premises at 35 Haymarket, 164 Piccadilly, 77-78 Strand, and 4 St Michaels Alley. In the design of these pharmacies, in the use of coloured leaded glass, English oak, granite, marble and bronze shopfronts, elaborate dispensing screens, sponge cases, and soda fountains, one finds the fullest expression of the early twentieth century pharmacy. The original business did not survive the depression and failed in 1931, continuing as Heppells (1932) Ltd. until later becoming part of Timothy Whites (pl. 98-107).

By contrast, in the nineteenth century small pharmacies could be established on a very small capital: as little as 6/6d in one exceptional case, a cash drug-store in a mining town, which claimed to have made-up 5,000 prescriptions in 16 months. The book *Opening a Pharmacy*, published in 1901 by *The Chemist and Druggist* assumed a starting capital of £400 in fitting-out, which was the sum John Bell had expended over 100 years earlier for the same purpose.

Many high-class pharmacies, including some of the "historic houses" such as John Bell & Co. retained, indeed cultivated, a deliberately archaic appearance (for the front-shop at least). This was readily acknowledged and often commented upon, as in the case of Cooper & Co. of Sloane Street, "Mr Cooper does not believe in displaying goods in his shop window; the emblems of his craft sufficing, with his reputation, for business purposes", and Dinneford's of New Bond Street, "The fittings are not in the newest style, but are splendid examples of an age when shop-fittings were intended not only to impress customers, but to last for a century". John Bell's front-shop was remodelled in 1824 by Theophilus Redwood, then an assistant with the firm. It remained a simple double shop without showcases or special dispensing arrangements until its closure in 1909 (pl. 86). Behind the scenes, however, the "elaboratory" was totally rebuilt in the late 1850s by John A. Godfrey, when it was fitted as a pharmaceutical manufacturing plant capable of making everything except chemicals on a large scale (pl. 87-88).

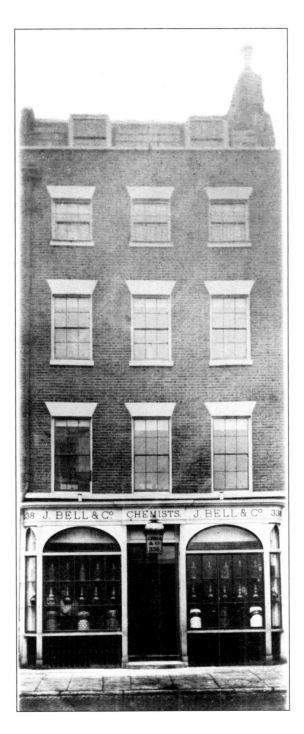

Plate 85.
John Bell & Co. Chemists, 338 Oxford Street, London, c. 1870.

John Bell's pharmacy, established at 338 Oxford Street in 1798, was not altered externally after the front was completely rebuilt in 1806. In most other pharmacies alterations of this kind were in turn succeeded by larger plate-glass windows, until, in order to maximise the attraction of the window display, the area of glass ran from ground to ceiling.

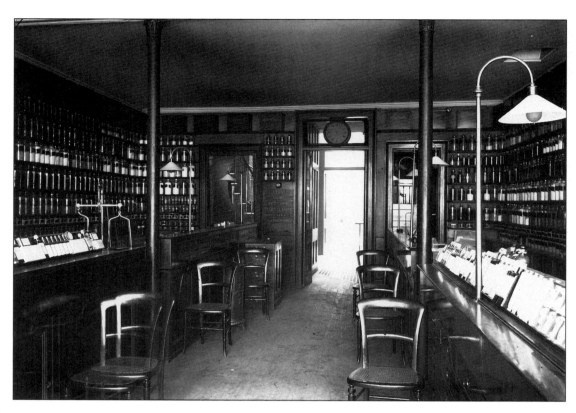

Plate 86.
The front-shop of John Bell & Co. as redesigned by Theophilus Redwood in 1824, c. 1900.

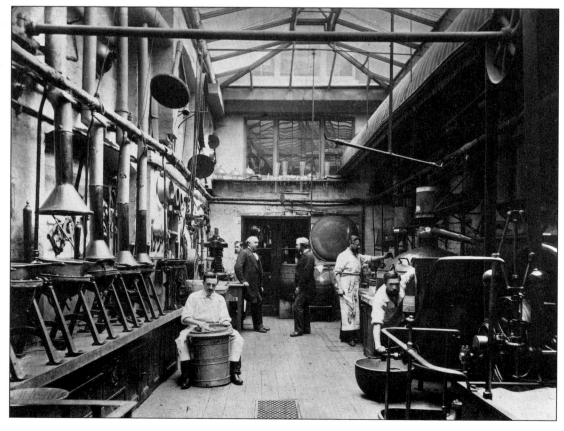

Plate 87.
John Bell & Co., 338 Oxford Street, London W1, 1871.

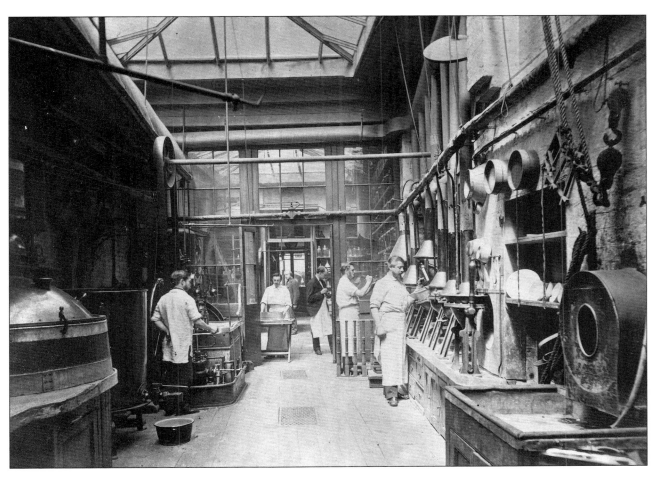

Plate 88.
John Bell & Co., 338 Oxford Street, London Wl, 1871.

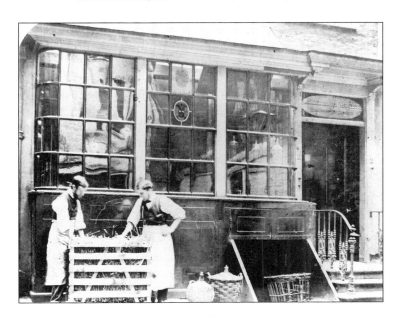

Plate 89.
The exterior of the old building of Allen & Hanbury's pharmacy, 2 Plough Court, London,
after the modernisations of 1856 and before its demolition in 1873.

Comparable pharmacies to John Bell & Co., with equally,
or more ancient buildings, such as Squire's and Allen and
Hanbury's, were extensively, though sometimes reluctantly,
rebuilt either because of town development, for expansion, or
to be perceived as "up to date".

50

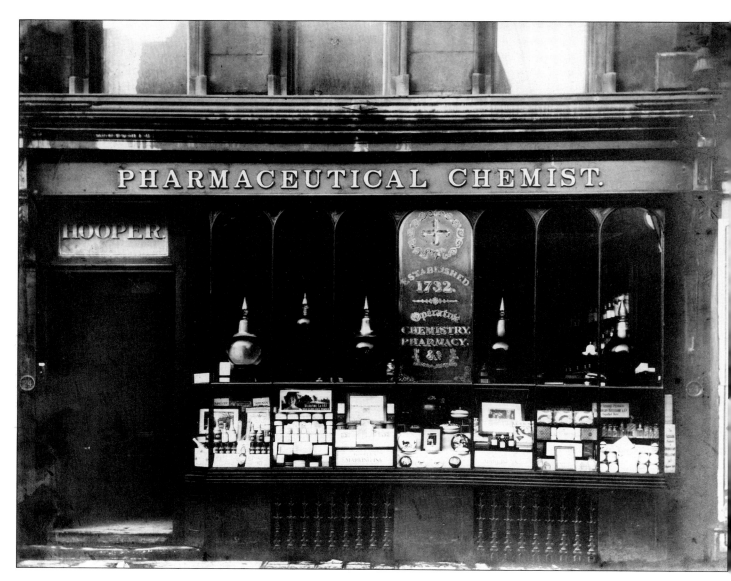

Plate 90.
The shopfront of William Hooper & Co., 24 Russell Street, Covent Garden, London, c. 1900.

The pharmacy of William Hooper & Co., 24 Russell Street, Covent Garden was established in 1732, and the building was one of the oldest continuously occupied pharmacies in London until its demolition in 1908. The business had associations with many famous medical men, including Dr Robert James (1703-1776), John Hunter (1728-1793), and Dr Thomas Percival (1740-1804). The shopfront was raised and plate-glass was fitted by Hooper in the 1840s, while retaining the ancient signboard with the sign of the red cross. Hooper had a reputation for concentrated infusions, galenical preparations and marking ink, but, near Drury Lane the theatrical trade was also important and in his shop it was reported that: "One sees the giant puff-boxes which tell of a more extensive area than the face to beautify".

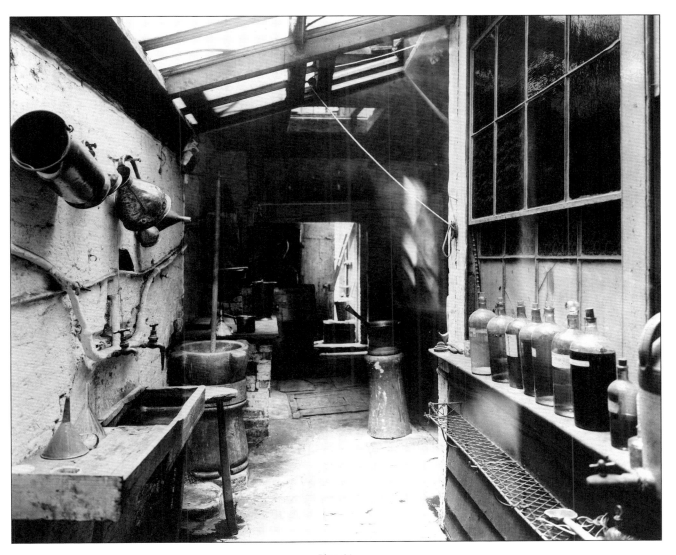

Plate 91.
The laboratory of William Hooper & Co., 24 Russell Street, Covent Garden, London, c. 1908.

Hooper's laboratory retained much of its original appearance.
Visible in the background are bell metal and marble mortars
and the splendid, much repaired, 60 gallon still of eighteenth
century pattern.

52

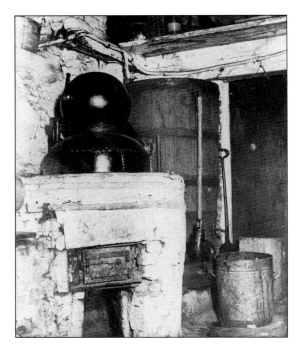

Plate 92.
Detail of the much-repaired 60 gallon still at 24 Russell Street, c. 1900.

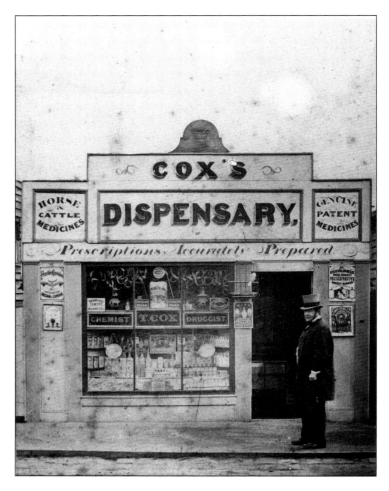

Plate 93.
The small dispensary of T. Cox at 35 Trumpington Street, Cambridge, before 1876.

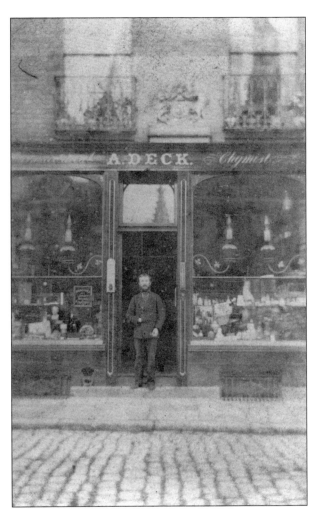

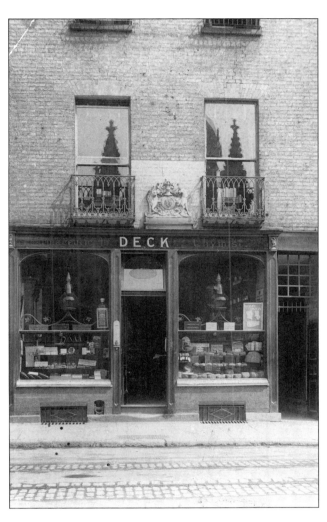

Plate 94.
A. Deck Chymist, 9 King's Parade, Cambridge, 1872.

Plate 95.
Deck Pharmaceutical Chymist, 9 King's Parade, Cambridge, c.1899.

Deck's pharmacy at 9 King's Parade, Cambridge is an
interesting example of a small pharmacy which retained its
shop-front completely unchanged for over 60 years. The
photograph of 1872 is the earliest amateur shot in the collection,
and probably the oldest actually taken by a pharmacist: W.I.
Pashler, chemist at the Addenbrookes Hospital.

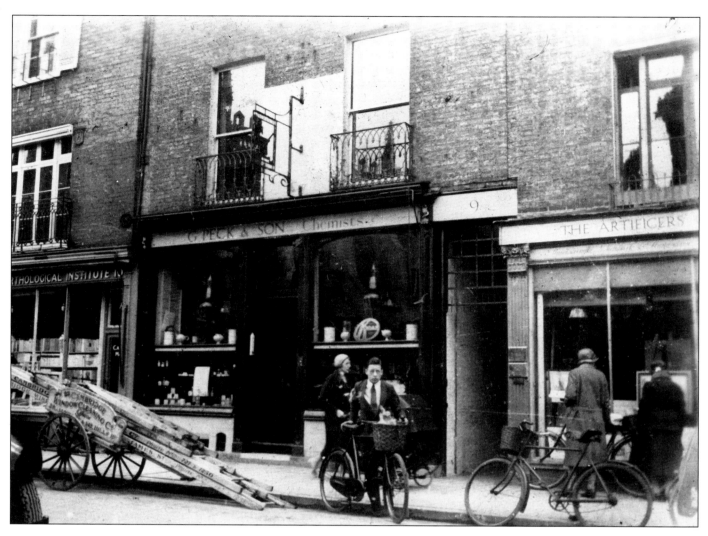

Plate 96.
G. Peck & Son, Chemists, 9 King's Parade, Cambridge, 1920s.

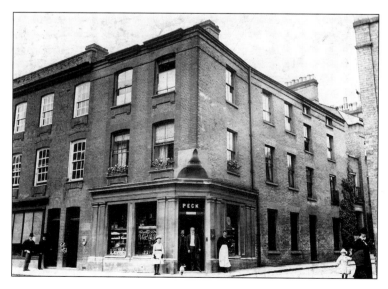

Plate 97.
G. Peck, 30 Trumpington Street, Cambridge, c. 1890.

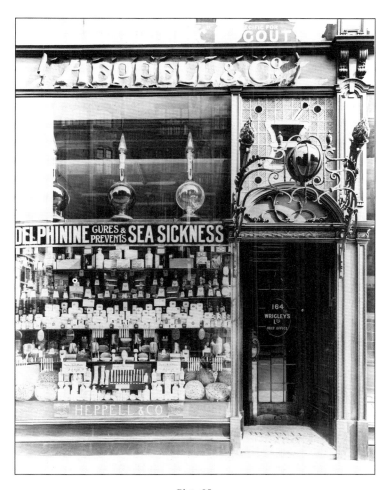

Plate 98.
The exterior of Heppel & Co., 164 Piccadilly, London, 1912.

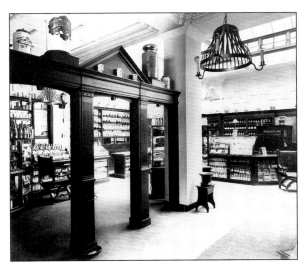

Plate 99.
The dispensing area of Heppel & Co., 164 Piccadilly, London, 1912.

The astonishing premises at 164 Piccadilly were finished in an idiosyncratic "Jacobean" style that was said to be a speciality of the architect, Mr Jennings (pl. 98). The inconveniently narrow frontage, only nine feet wide, was compensated for by a spacious hallway which led to the dispensing department. Here, tinned iron "electroliers", like some ancient instruments of torture, were suspended from the ceiling (pl. 99). The dispensary, furnished with an old English oak settle, must have been one of the most lavish ever built. The remarkable fireplace, constructed of eighteenth century brick, was decorated with an ambitious fresco painted by Mildred Jennings (pl. 100). It was said approvingly that: "Evidences of business are present but are not intrusive, yet tempt one to buy". The premises at 164 Piccadilly were specialists in perfume and toiletries, and "Kings and other Royal personages... have visited the pharmacy when they have been staying at the Ritz Hotel... and many of them have expressed their delight at the artistic furnishing of the place".

56

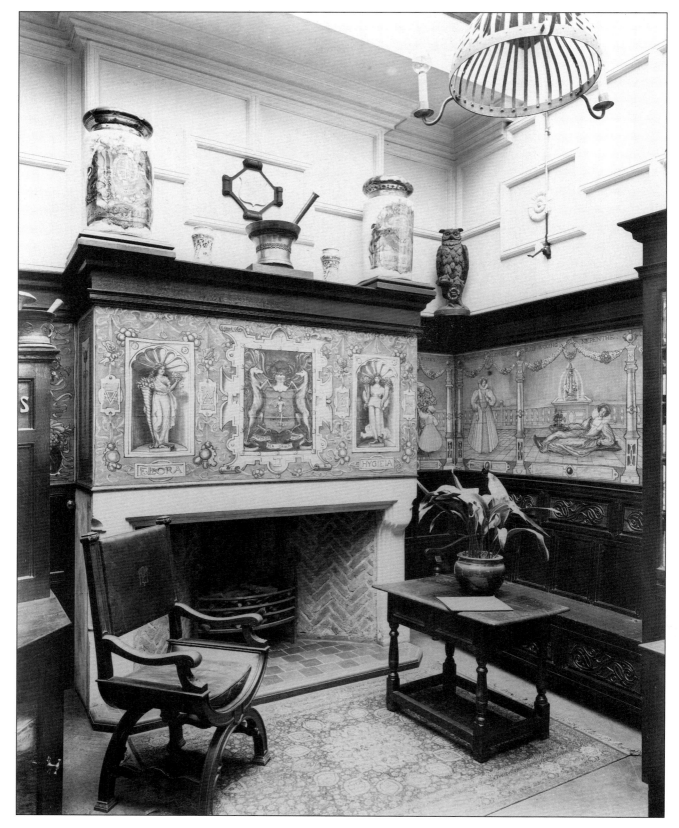

Plate 100.
Heppel & Co., 164 Piccadilly, London, 1912.

57

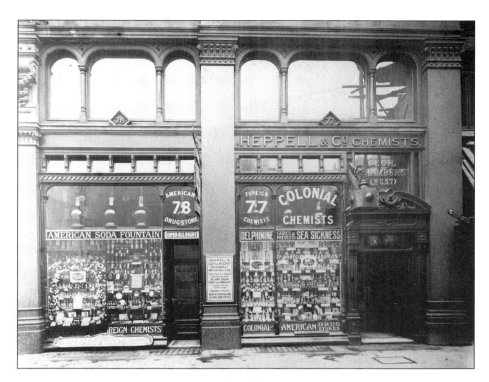

Plate 101.
Heppel & Co. Chemists, 77-78 Strand, London, 1912.

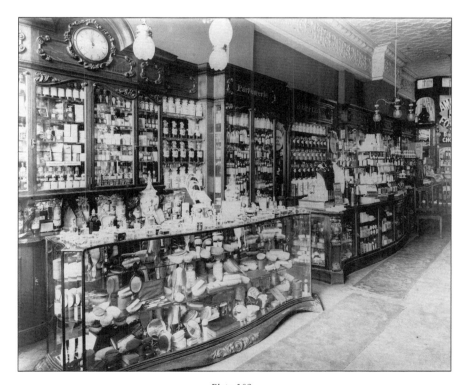

Plate 102.
Heppel & Co. Chemists, Hotel Cecil Buildings, 77-78 Strand, London, 1912.

The Hotel Cecil branch at 77-78 Strand opened in the early years of the century and was distinctly American in character (pl. 101-103). Note the sign above the counter urging customers to "drink Coca-Cola" (Heppels was also associated with the introduction of Wrigley's spearmint "Pepsin" gum from the USA at this time). The wonderfully atmospheric interior shot, taken by gaslight, illustrates another notable feature - namely that the businesses were originally worked by a double staff, so as to provide an all-night service. Later this branch was "only" open from 6.00 in the morning until 12.30 at night. It is plain why the firm chose an owl with illuminated eyes as its symbol (pl. 105).

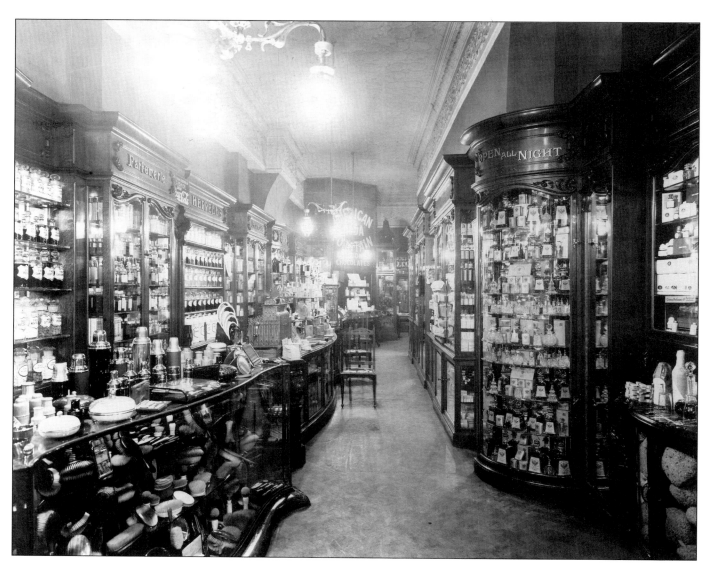

Plate 103.
Heppel & Co. Chemists, Hotel Cecil Buildings, 77-78 Strand, London, 1912.

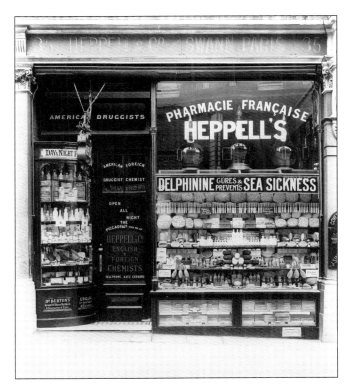

Plate 104.
Exterior of Heppel & Co. Pharmacie Française, 35 Haymarket, London, 1912.

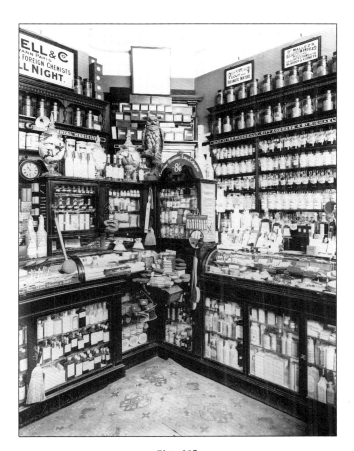

Plate 105.
Interior of Heppel & Co. Pharmacie Française, 35 Haymarket, London, 1912.

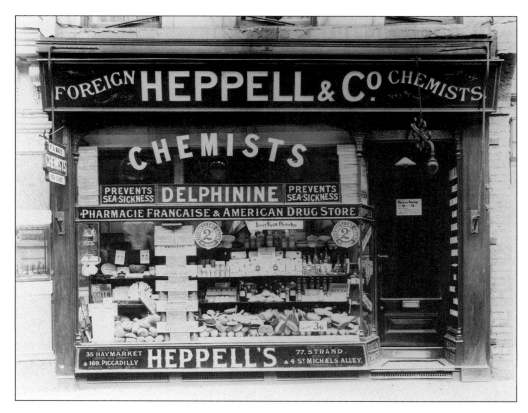

Plate 106.
Exterior of Heppel & Co., 4 St Michaels Alley, 1912.

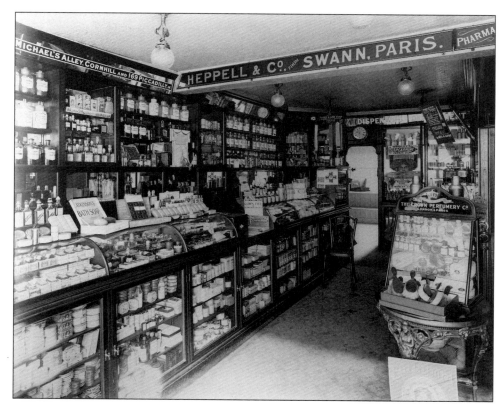

Plate 107.
Interior of Heppel & Co., 4 St Michaels Alley, 1912.

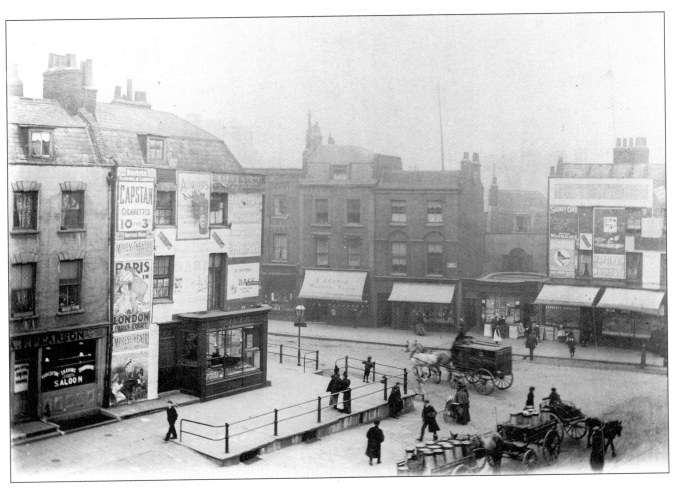

Plate 108.
Cross Street and Essex Road corner, Islington, London, opposite to the Wallis pharmacy, 1903.

The appearance of the small corner shop of J.T.W. Wallis, and its urban setting at 78 Essex Road, Islington, is preserved in a number of fine amateur photographs taken by T.E. Wallis and his brother between 1895 and 1902. The distinctive appearance of even a small pharmacy with its large carboys and coloured lamp can be contrasted with the other shops in this part of Islington in Wallis' townscape (pl. 108). In addition to several views of the rather gloomy interior of their father's pharmacy, a darkness not solely due to underexposure of the negative, Wallis most unusually photographed the family drawing room as part of this series, thereby providing a rare glimpse of life "above the shop".

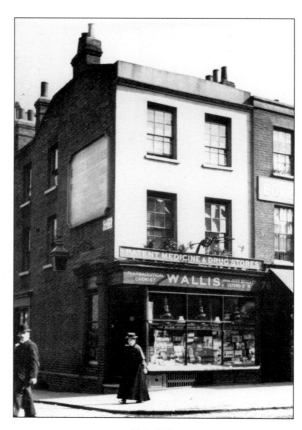

Plate 109.
"Charlie's photo of father's shop". Wallis Pharmaceutical Chemist patent medicine & drug stores, 78 Essex Road, Islington, 1895.

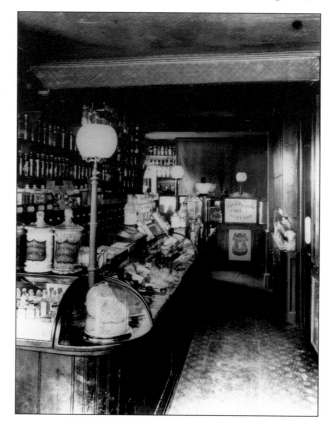

Plate 110.
78 Essex Road counter, the interior of Wallis Pharmaceutical Chemist patent medicine & drug stores, 1902.

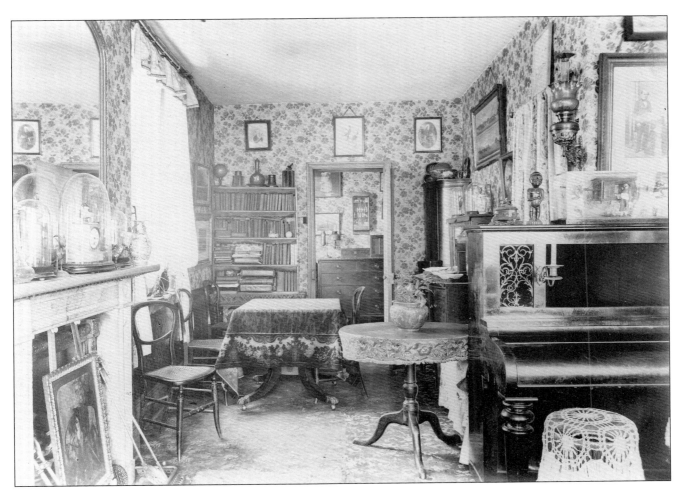

Plate 111.
Above the shop at 78 Essex Road, 1902.

64

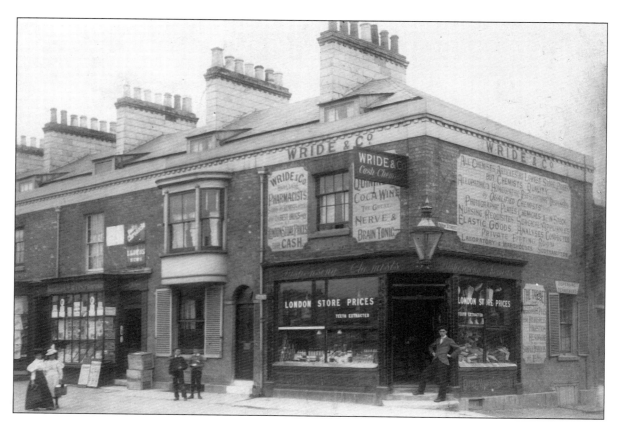

Plate 112.
An early multiple store: Wride & Co., 34 High Street, Shirley, Hampshire, c.1880-1890.

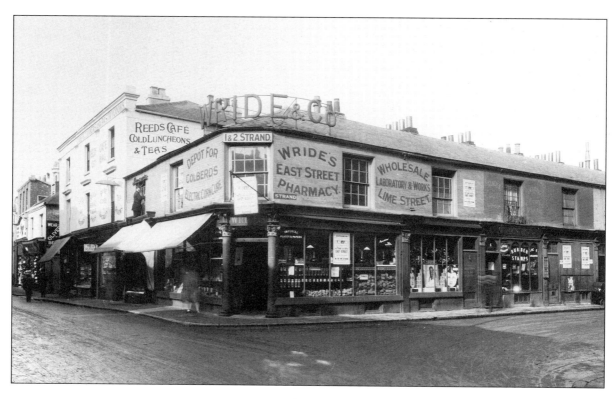

Plate 113.
The original premises of Wride & Co., at 1-2 The Strand, East Street, Southampton, prior to demolition in 1929.

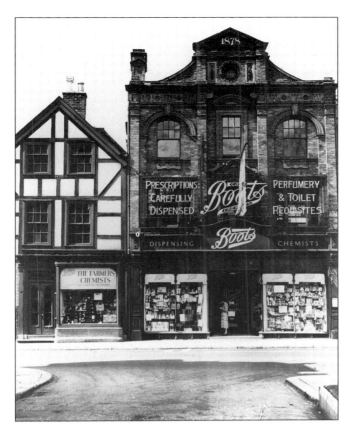

Plate 114.
Boots dispensing chemists, 10-11 Market Square, Stafford, 1950s.

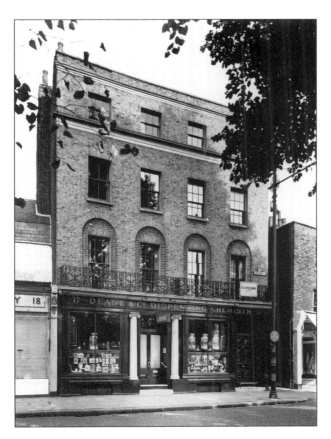

Plate 115.
Deane & Co. dispensing chemists, 17 The Pavement, Clapham, London, October 1953.

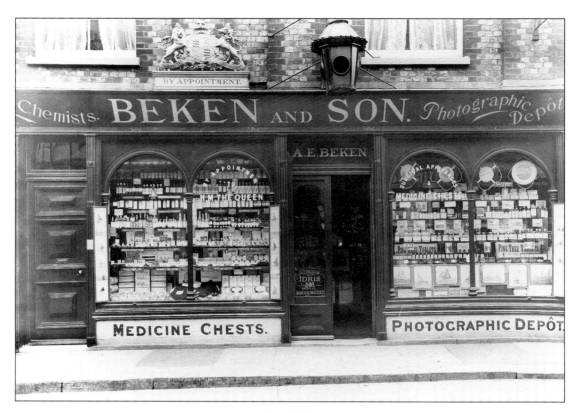

Plate 116.
Beken & Son Chemists, Cowes, Isle of Wight, c. 1900.

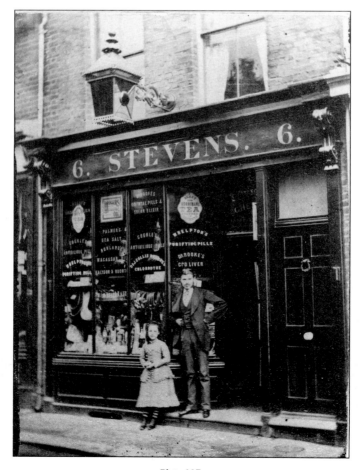

Plate 117.
James Stevens with his daughter, probably on the opening of his pharmacy,
6 High Street, New Brompton (Gillingham), 1872.

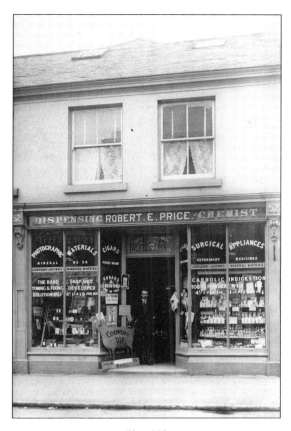

Plate 118.
Robert E. Price Dispensing Chemist, 72 High Street, Rhyl, 1909.

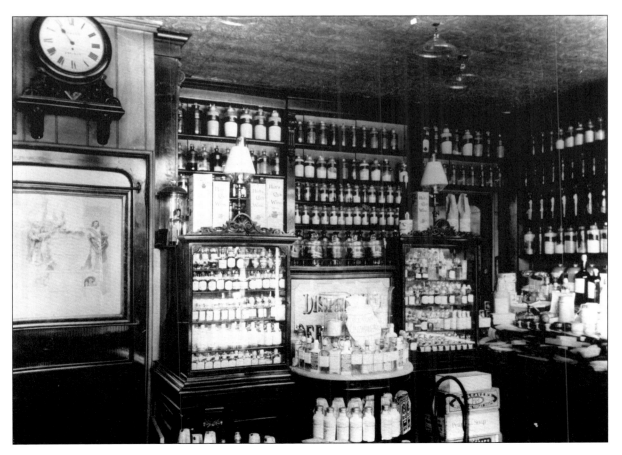

Plate 119.
Pharmacy in Enfield Town: Successor to John Tuff, Enfield, Middlesex, c. 1898-1918.

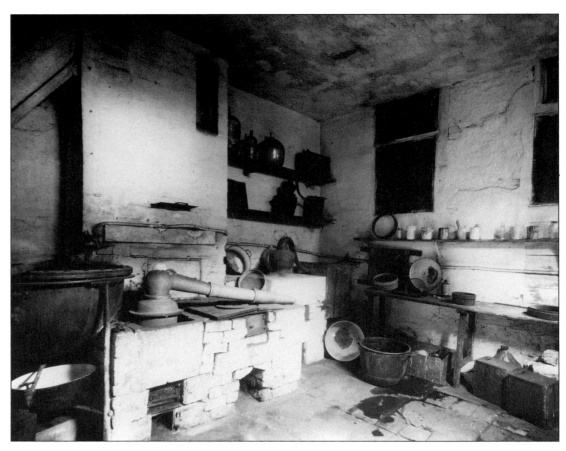

Plate 120.
Boilerhouse and laboratory in the pharmacy of Nathaniel Smith, 373 High Street, Cheltenham, Gloucester, c. 1900.

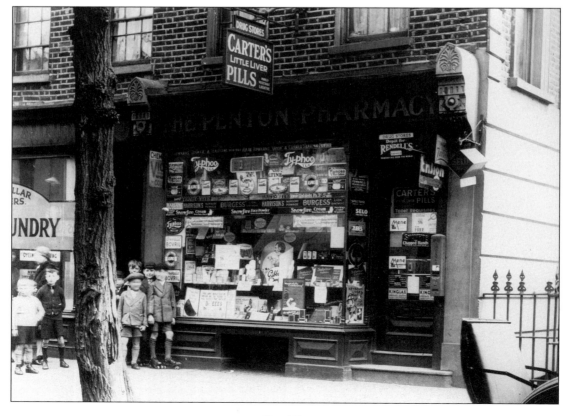

Plate 121.
The Penton Pharmacy, London, c. 1930.

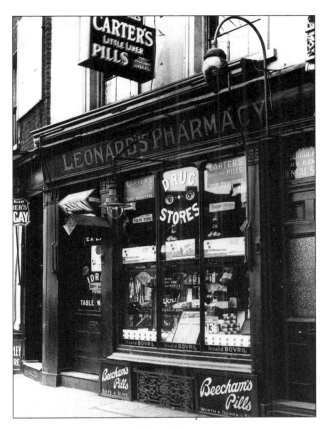

Plate 122.
Leonard's Pharmacy, London, c. 1930.

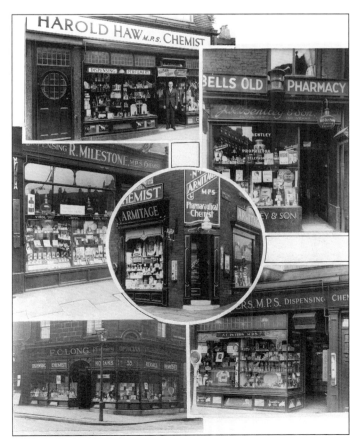

Plate 123.
Retail establishments in Leeds, 1934.

70

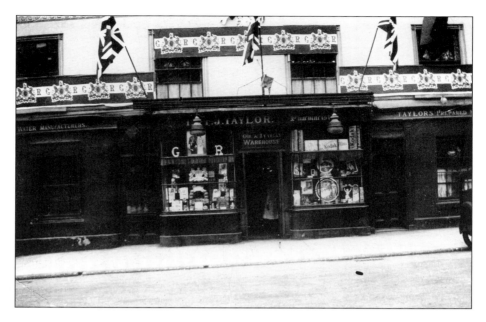

Plate 124.
The exterior of T. & F. J. Taylor Pharmacists, 36 High Street, Newport Pagnell, 1935.

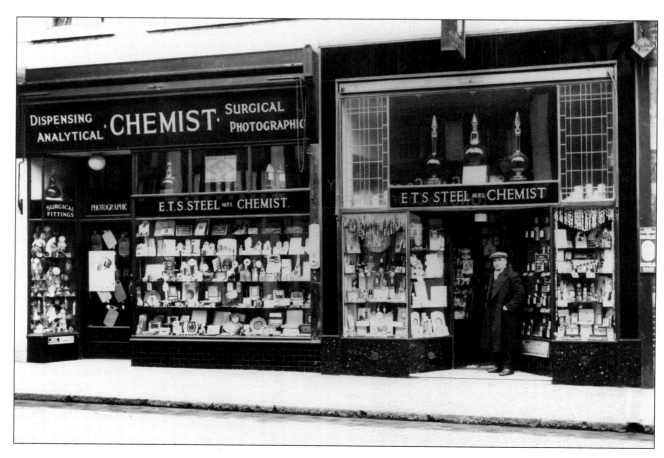

Plate 125.
"The manner in which two existing shopfronts have been linked":
The pharmacy of E.T.S. Steel, 58-59 East Street, Southampton, 1939.

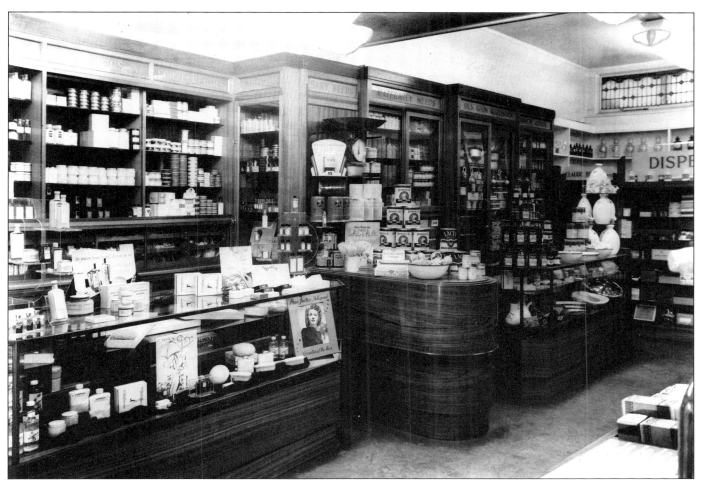

Plate 126.
Claude Benton Ltd., Norwich, c. 1950.

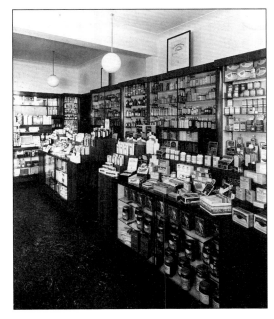

Plate 127.
Gordon Smith, MPS, dispensing chemist of
Ashley Road, Hale, Cheshire, 1938.

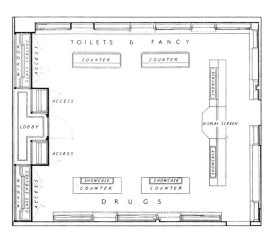

Shop plan and counter layout, Gordon Smith MPS, Hale, Cheshire.

72

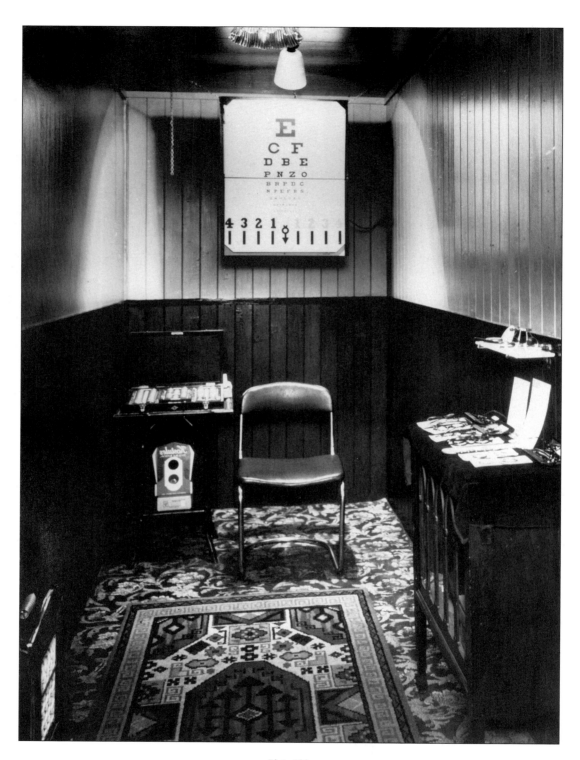

Plate 128.
The new eye-test room and equipment at Forster, Chemist Optician,
11 Faircross Parade, New Barking, Essex, 1930s.

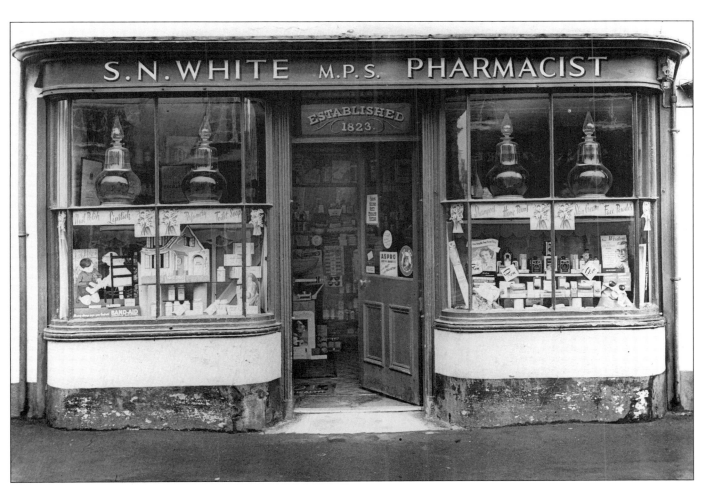

Plate 129.
S.N. White, The Pharmacy, Topsham, Devon, c. 1953.

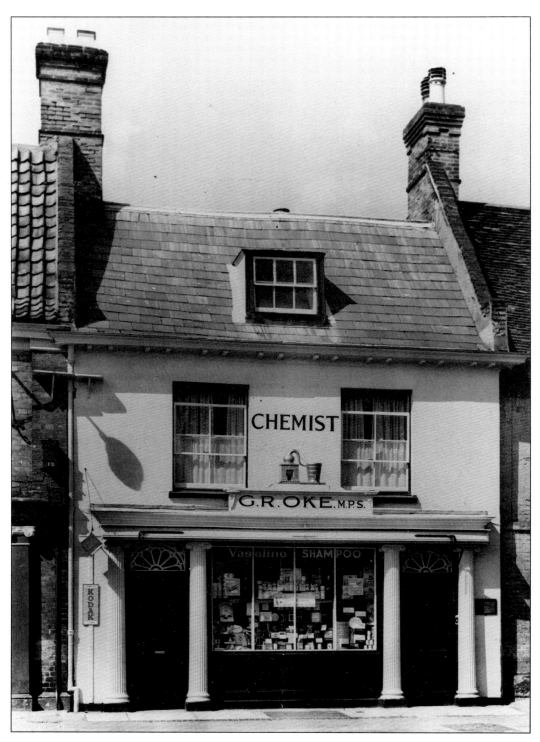

Plate 130.
The exterior of G. R. Oke, 14 Market Place, Aylsham, Norfolk, 1953.

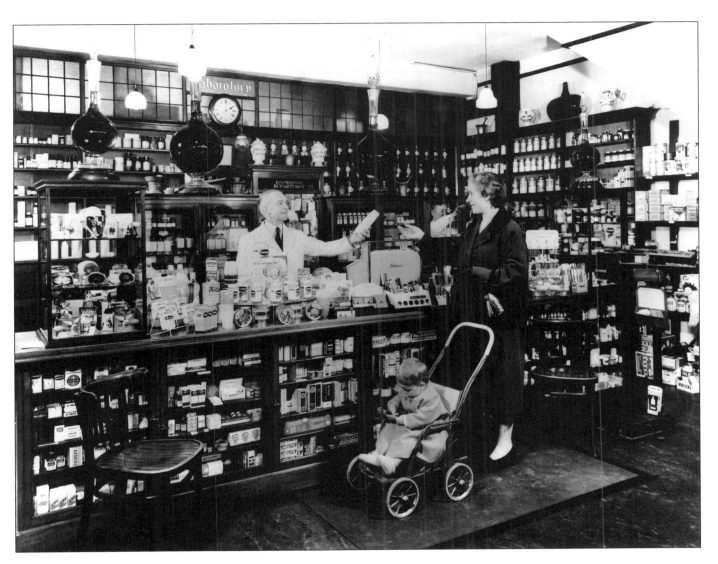

Plate 131.
"The Pharmacist in retail practice". The interior of the pharmacy of R. J. Mellowes,
20 Bush Hill Parade, Enfield, Middlesex, 1959.

76

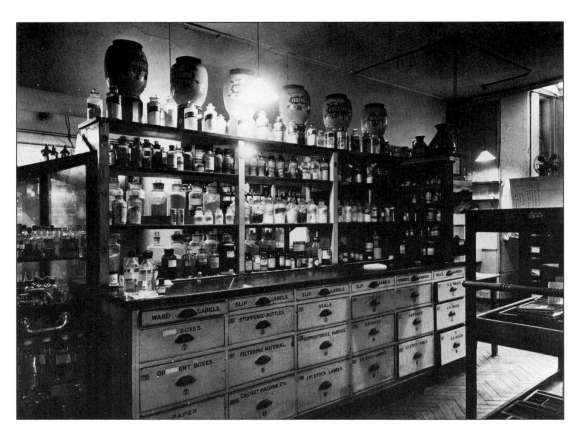

Plate 132.
The pharmacy department, St George's Hospital, London, c. 1950.

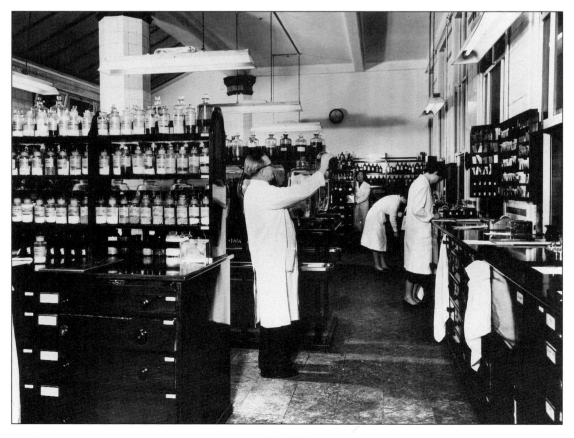

Plate 133.
"The Pharmacist in hospital: the dispensary", St Bartholomew's Hospital, London, 1959.

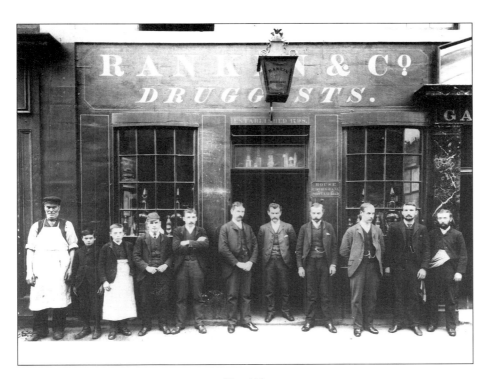

Plate 134.
The staff of Rankin & Co. Druggists, 7 King Street, Kilmarnock, c.1890.

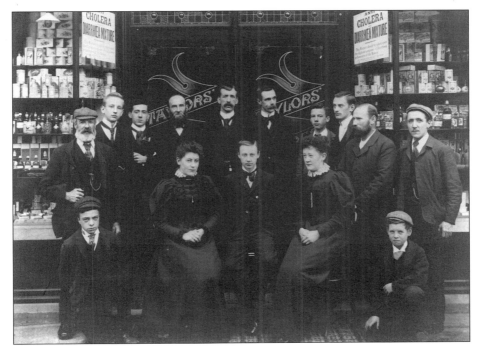

Plate 135.
The staff of Taylors' Drug Co. Ltd., 16 Beulah Street to 54 Station Parade, Harrogate, c. 1900.

The impressive appearance of many nineteenth century pharmacies was only maintained through the hard work and long hours of a large establishment consisting of pharmacists, assistants, apprentices, carters, errand boys, laboratory and manufacturing staff. Quite how large is shown by several group photographs. The cleaning and extensive window dressing of the pharmacy was done by the assistants, and even the most elaborate displays were often changed weekly.

# SOCIAL SETTING

The major part of the Society's collections records an "official" or public face of pharmacy. Yet a small group of photographs provide a glimpse of the other side to this professional world.

In certain cases, the survival of these images appears to be due to an amateur interest in photography fostered through pharmacy. Pictures of family groups, domestic interiors and topographical snapshots reveal details of life "above the shop", most fully exemplified by the album compiled by Dr T.E. Wallis of both his domestic and working environment (see pl. 108-111).

An unusual shot portrays Mr John Buxton Payne and his daughters playing billiards. Payne began his career as a chemist and druggist who set up a photographic business in Piccadilly, Manchester. In 1880 he moved to Newcastle to join the firm of Mawson and Swan as assistant to Sir Joseph Wilson Swan, collaborating in many projects concerned with the development of photography and the electric light.

Other shots show a variety of social events. For instance, two charabanc parties of employees from John Bell, Hills & Lucas Ltd. pose for their group photographs on the corner of the Old Kent Road, in East London (pl.137-138). By contrast Mrs John Attfield is shown at a more genteel occasion, surrounded by over 250 guests at a garden party to mark the retirement of her husband as professor to the School of Pharmacy (pl. 139). As a major social event of the pharmaceutical world, a detailed account of the party, the speeches, its guest list, the menu and even the musical accompaniment was reproduced in the pharmaceutical press of July 1897. Dr John Attfield FRS, standing to the right of the table, was a leading figure in pharmacy for more than three decades, particularly noted for his contribution to pharmaceutical education and to the establishment of the British Pharmaceutical Conference. Originally apprenticed to a manufacturing chemist, he subsequently studied at the Society's School where in 1862 he was appointed Director and Demonstrator in Chemistry and Pharmacy, a title later changed to Professor of Practical Chemistry. His retirement celebration, as described in *The Pharmaceutical Journal*, culminated in the presentation of an exceptionally elaborate gift: "an illuminated autograph album (containing 1,214 signatures of friends and pupils) in a polished oak casket, together with a silver tray and silver tea and coffee service".

A series of delightful albums entitled *Pharmacists at Play* record an annual sporting competition organised for Pharmaceutical Associations in the London area (pl. 140-142). Teams representing the Associations competed for the Maw Challenge Shield in a variety of events; tennis, golf, bowls, croquet, putting and quoits. The competition was held at the Maws sports ground, Monken Hadley Estate, New Barnet over two days. A military band and a marquee for refreshments added to the lighthearted atmosphere of the occasion.

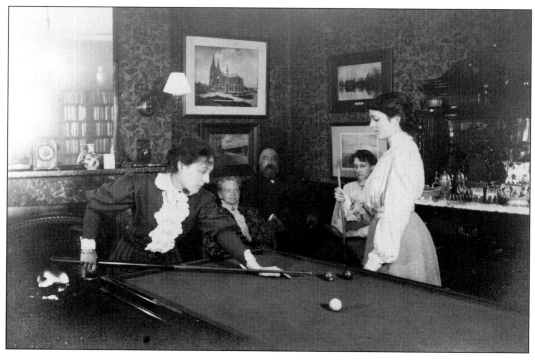

Plate 136.
The Payne family, Newcastle-upon-Tyne, Northumberland, 1890s.

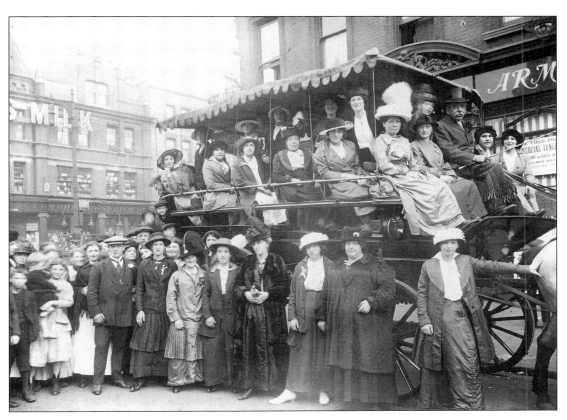

Plate 137.
John Bell, Hills & Lucas Ltd., staff outing, 29 September 1919.

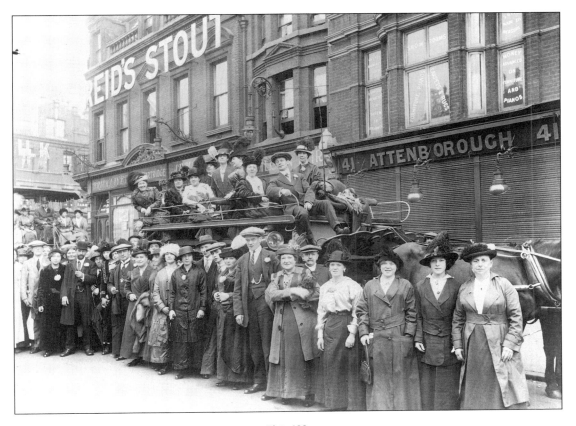

Plate 138.
John Bell, Hills & Lucas Ltd., staff outing, 1919.

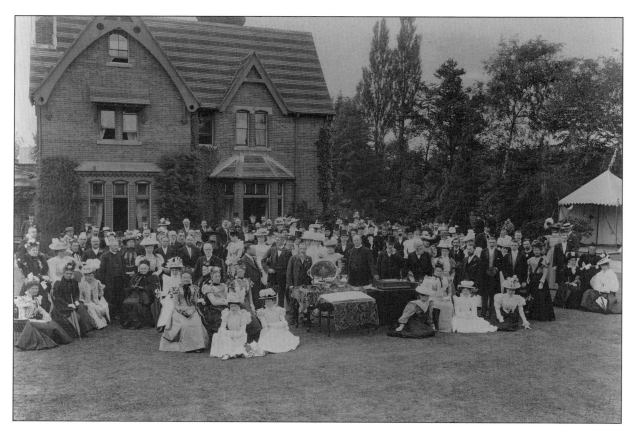

Plate 139.
Mrs Attfield at home, Ashlands, Watford, Hertfordshire, 10 July 1897.

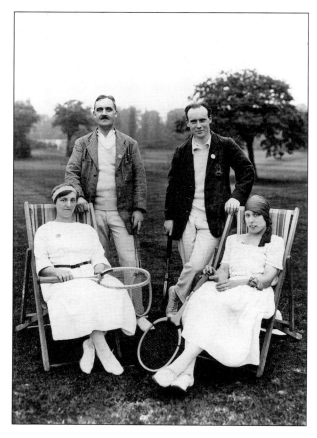

Plate 140.
Maw challenge shield competition, New Barnet, 1925.

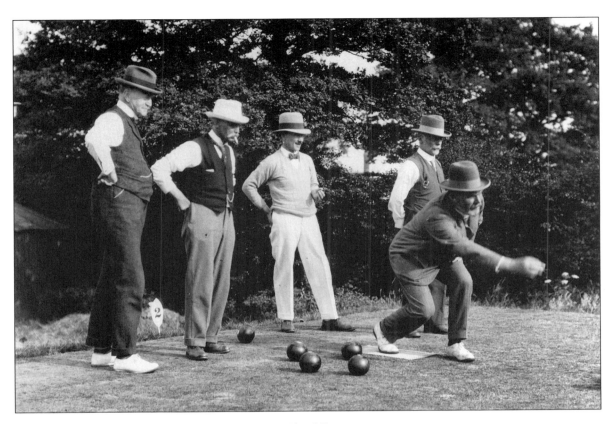

Plate 141.
Maw challenge shield competition, New Barnet, 1925.

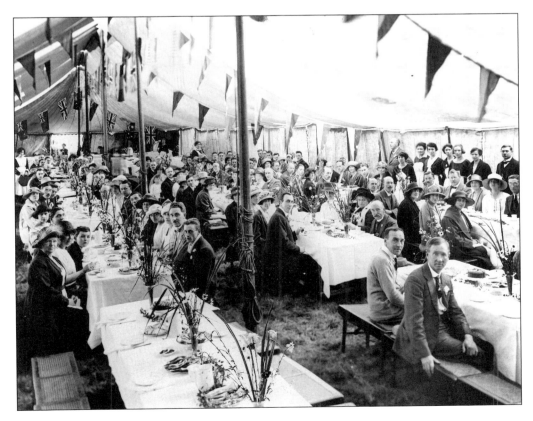

Plate 142.
Maw challenge shield competition, New Barnet, 1923.

# PHARMACEUTICAL RAW MATERIALS AND PRODUCTION

Among the collection's earliest images are those which record the production of pharmaceutical raw materials.

The cultivation of quinine is the subject of a remarkable collection of photographs from the archive of John Eliot Howard, an authority on the *cinchona* species and their alkaloids. Derived from the bark of the cinchona plant and used in the treatment of malaria, it was one of the most important and valuable drugs available in the nineteenth century.

A snapshot of a picnic at Coroico in the Yungas, an area which produced the best bark in Bolivia, provides a rare view of cinchona cultivation in its native continent in 1882 (pl. 143). The plantation belonged to Manuel Calderon, a friend and correspondent of Charles Ledger. Over 30 years earlier, Ledger (who is recognised for having discovered and introduced the purest species of cinchona yet known to the West) had encouraged Calderon to sow cinchona seed on this estate.

A photograph, dated 1861, of the propagating house at Ootacamund, India, shows the experimental cultivation of the young cinchona plants collected by C.R. Markham and Richard Spruce (pl. 145). These British Government gardens and plantations became a major centre for producing cinchona during the second half of the nineteenth century.

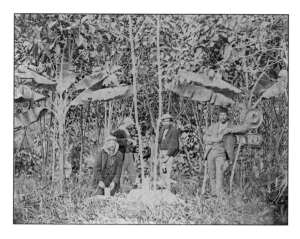

Plate 143.
View of San Carlos cinchona plantation
with the proprietor Señor Don Manuel Calderon, Bolivia,
20 December 1882.

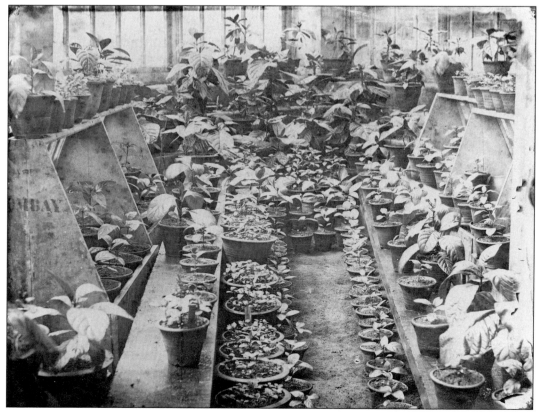

Plate 144.
View of cinchona plants in the propagating house at the Government gardens Ootacamund, Madras, India, 9 September 1861.

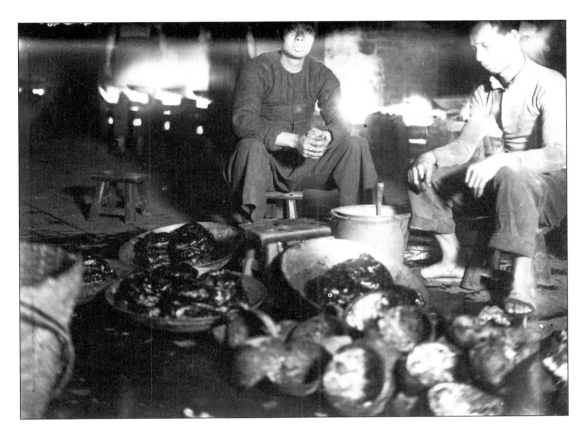

Plate 145.
Smoking opium production at the Government Monopoly Factory, Hong Kong, 1915.

By 1900 the use of opium was subject to much stricter legal and medical control in Britain than it had been half a century earlier. It had largely been replaced as the medically prescribed treatment for insomnia and fevers by alternatives such as chloral, quinine and the bromides. Nevertheless, opium as a constituent of many popular brands of proprietary self medication continued to be consumed in substantial quantities.

Opium addiction remained a chronic problem in many parts of the World, particularly in the Far East during the first decades of this century, in spite of various international attempts to limit its production and trade through measures agreed by the International Opium Commission, the Treaty of Versailles and the League of Nations. In Hong Kong, for instance, opium continued to be imported from India, Turkey and Persia. Consumption increased, even though the drug was controlled by a government monopoly and attempts were made to limit its use by the closure of opium dens.

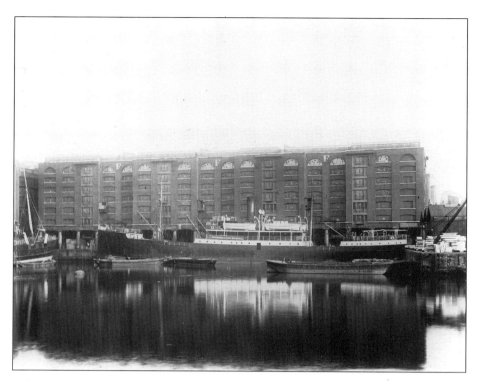

Plate 146.
Exterior of the rubber warehouse and facilities of the Argos Steamship Co.,
London & Bremen Line, St Katherine's docks, with moored freighter, c. 1910.

The expansion of large-scale trade in pharmaceutical raw materials during the nineteenth century was not only confined to crude drugs of plant origin. Many materials had to be imported. Non-medicinal commodities used in the production of medical and pharmaceutical equipment and appliances, are illustrated by two views of the transportation and storage of rubber in the early twentieth century.

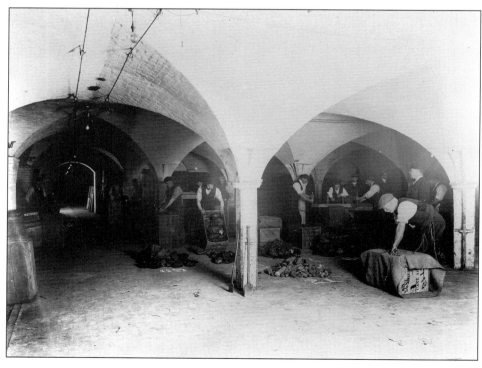

Plate 147.
Interior of the rubber vaults, St Katherine's docks, London, c. 1910.

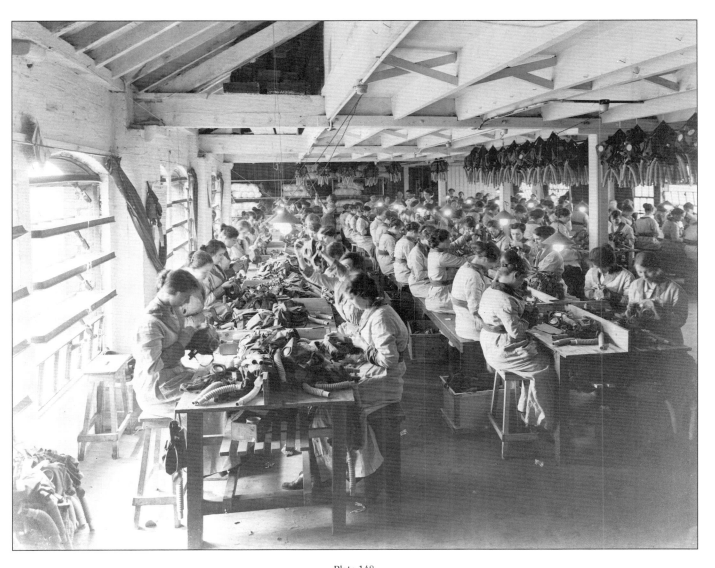

Plate 148.
"Antigas" work. Fitting-up box-respirator gas masks at the Oxford Works, Tower Bridge Road, c. 1917/1918.

Although primarily concerned with the wholesale and manufacturing side of pharmacy, the business of John Bell, Hills & Lucas & Co. turned its efforts to producing anti-gas respirators during the First World War, for which they engaged a large female workforce.

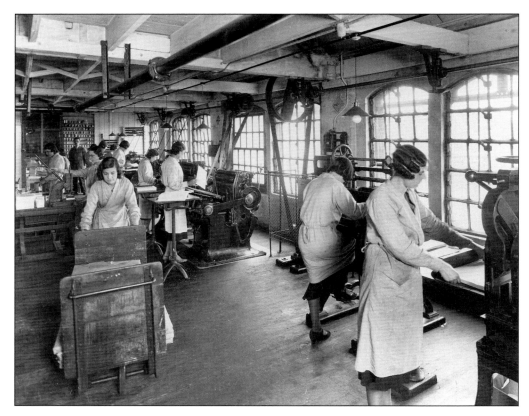

Plate 149.
Printing and labelling room, 1933.

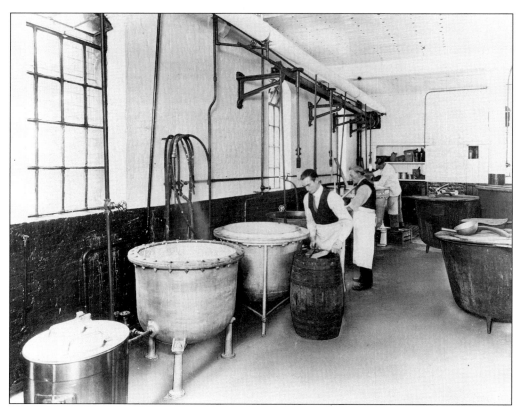

Plate 150.
Manufacturing plant, John Bell, Hills & Lucas, 1933.

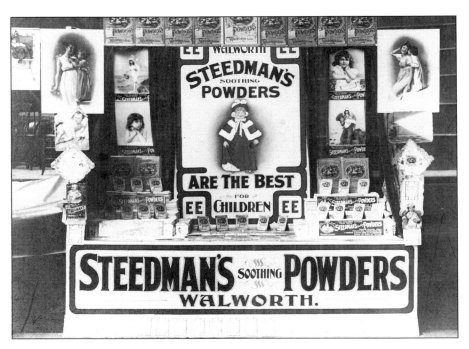

Plate 151.
Steedman's stall at a baby show, Derby, c. 1900.

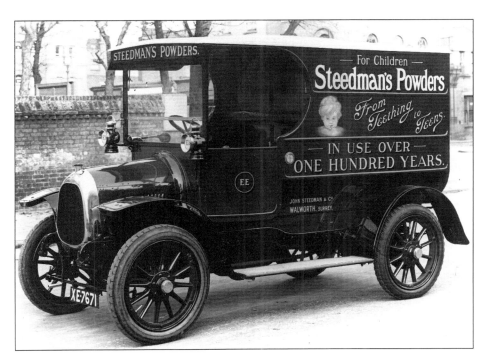

Plate 152.
Delivery van in Steedman's livery. The bodywork of 1913 adapted to a Beardmore chassis, 1922.

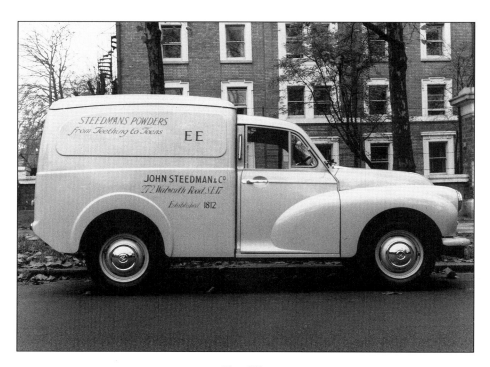

Plate 153.
Steedman's Morris delivery van, Walworth, Surrey, November 1956.

The pharmacy of John Steedman was established in 1812 from where he launched his business in trade name medicines. As John Steedman & Co. the firm was to become one of the best known proprietary medicine manufacturers of the nineteenth century, noted particularly for its "Children's Soothing Powders". This popular brand was still sold until the early 1950s when a link was finally established between the incidence of Pink disease and mercurial preparations.

The original formulations of Steedman's products were compounded in his Walworth pharmacy from where their reputation spread. A variety of advertising material was used to promote brand loyalty in a competitive market including a range of display cards and a series of advisory literature aimed at young mothers (pl. 151).

# ILLUSTRATIONS INDEX

**1.** "One of Mr Swan's earliest carbon prints". John Mawson, 1863. carbon print: possibly by Sir Joseph Wilson Swan.
**19.5 x 15cm (mounted). SZ.2265.**

**2.** Sir Joseph Wilson Swan, as president of the Newcastle-on-Tyne and Northern Counties Photographic Association, 1881. albumen print.
**9.5 x 13.8cm (mounted). SZ.5804.**

**3.** Headquarters of the Pharmaceutical Society of Great Britain 1841-1976, 17 Bloomsbury Square, London, 1883/4. albumen print: Martin & Sallnow, 416 Strand, London WC.
**15 x 20cm . SZ.829.**

**4.** The Pharmaceutical Society's house in the 1930s. gelatin print: Miles & Kaye Ltd., 100 Southampton Row, High Holborn, London WC1.
**29 x 25cm . SZ.850.**

**5.** Council chamber, second floor of 17 Bloomsbury Square, 1883/4. albumen print: Martin & Sallnow, 416 Strand, London WC.
**10 x 15cm (mounted). SZ.57.**

**6.** Council chamber, 17 Bloomsbury Square, 1892. gelatin print from a "Sandell" dry plate.
**28.5 x 37cm (mounted). SZ.2251.**

**7.** "Chemistry Museum", ground floor of 17 Bloomsbury Square, 1883/4. albumen print: unmarked but probably Martin & Sallnow.
**15 x 20.5cm (mounted). SZ.5.**

**8.** The museum, 29 November 1937. gelatin print.
**19.5 x 25cm . SZ.1783.**

**9.** Museum, 17 Bloomsbury Square, 1883/4. albumen print: unmarked but probably Martin & Sallnow.
**15 x 20.5cm (mounted). SZ.238.**

**10.** Museum, 17 Bloomsbury Square, 1931. gelatin print: R.B. Fleming & Co.
**16 x 21cm. SZ.1753.**

**11.** The library, and readers, 17 Bloomsbury Square, 1883/4. albumen print: Martin & Sallnow, 416 Strand, London WC.
**15 x 20cm (mounted). SZ.261.**

**12.** Library, 17 Bloomsbury Square, 1928. gelatin print.
**16 x 21cm (mounted). SZ.1742.**

**13.** The office staff, 1898, including from left to right: G.E. Jones, A.J. Chater, H. Froude, R. Bremridge, E.H. Lee, J.W. Knapman, W.H. Baker, and H. Moon. carbon print.
**16.5 x 21.5cm (mounted). SZ.3092.**

**14.** Passage in 72 Great Russell Street, 1905, the Pharmaceutical Journal's waiting room, taken for *The Chemists Annual*, 1906. gelatin print.
**24.5 x 19.5cm (mounted). SZ.75.**

**15.** Law department, ground floor, 16 Bloomsbury Square, October 1931. gelatin print: R.B. Fleming & Co.
**16 x 21cm. SZ.1731.**

**16.** Registry, 17 Bloomsbury Square, 1937. gelatin print: The "Topical" Press Agency Ltd., 10 & 11 Red Lion Court, Fleet Street, London, EC4.
**19.5 x 25.2cm. SZ.1750.**

**17.** Typists room on the third floor at the back of 16 Bloomsbury Square, 1931. gelatin print: R.B. Fleming & Co.
**16 x 21cm. SZ.1732.**

**18.** Jacob Bell as editor of *The Pharmaceutical Journal*, 1891 from a daguerreotype of the mid 1840s. albumen copy print: Barrauds Ltd., 263 Oxford Street W (Regent Circus), London.
**13.5 x 10cm. SZ.6000.**

**19.** Jacob Bell, founder of the Pharmaceutical Society of Great Britain, c. 1852. daguerreotype, plate stamped: 20, Mayall; case stamped: (Obv.) By Appointment Mr Kilburn, 234 Regent Street, (Rev.) 224 Regent Street, J.E. Mayall, Daguerreotype Institution, 433 West Strand.
**13 x 10cm (quarter plate, cased). SZ.1000.**

**20.** Thomas Hyde Hills, successor to the firm of John Bell & Co., in humorous mood, c.1867. albumen print, *carte-de-visite:* W. Walker & Sons, 64 Margaret Street, Cavendish Square, London.
**8.8 x 5.7cm (mounted in album). SZ.1502.**

**21.** George Webb Sandford, c.1867. albumen print, *carte-de-visite:* Maull & Co., 187a Piccadilly W, 62 Cheapside EC, Tavistock House, Fulham Road, London.
**9.1 x 5.8cm (mounted in album). SZ.1507.**

**22.** William L. Bird, c.1867. albumen print, *carte-de-visite:* W. Walker & Sons, 64 Margaret Street, Cavendish Square, London.
**8.8 x 5.7cm (mounted in album). SZ.1515.**

**23.** George Meggeson, c.1864. albumen print, *carte-de-visite:* Horne & Thornthwaite, 121, 122, 123, Newgate Street, London.
**9.2 x 5.8cm (mounted in album). SZ.1516.**

**24.** George Waugh, c.1865. albumen print: Maull & Co., 62 Cheapside EC, 187 Piccadilly & Tavistock House, Fulham Road, London.
**20 x 15cm (mounted). SZ.505.**

**25.** Thomas Standring, c.1865. albumen print: Maull & Co., 62 Cheapside EC, 187 Piccadilly & Tavistock House, Fulham Road, London.
**20 x 15cm (mounted). SZ.506.**

**26.** Henry Deane, c.1865. albumen print: Maull & Co., 62 Cheapside EC, 187 Piccadilly & Tavistock House, Fulham Road, London.
**20 x 15cm (mounted). SZ.535.**

**27.** Peter Squire, c.1860. albumen print, *carte-de-visite:* Nadar, photographie du Grand Hotel, 35 Boulevart des Capucines, Paris.
**8.8 x 5.7cm (mounted in album). SZ.1534.**

**28.** Peter Squire, c.1865. albumen print: Maull & Co., 62 Cheapside EC, 187 Piccadilly & Tavistock House, Fulham Road, London.
**20 x 15cm (mounted). SZ.510.**

**29.** Thomas N.R. Morson, c.1865. albumen print: Maull & Co., 62 Cheapside EC, 187 Piccadilly & Tavistock House, Fulham Road, London.
**20 x 15cm (mounted). SZ.519.**

**30.** Augustus Bird, c.1865. albumen print: Maull & Co., 62 Cheapside EC, 187 Piccadilly & Tavistock House, Fulham Road, London.
**20 x 15cm (mounted). SZ.541.**

**31.** Professor Theophilus Redwood, c.1870. albumen print.
**25 x 20.5cm (mounted). SZ.654.**

**32.** William Martindale, 1879. albumen print: Maull & Fox, 187a Piccadilly, London.
**20 x 15cm (mounted). SZ.547.**

**33.** Dr William A. Tilden, 1872. albumen print: Maull & Co., 187a, Piccadilly & 62 Cheapside, London.
**20 x 15cm (mounted). SZ.507.**

**34.** A Pharmaceutical Society Council dinner at the Holborn Restaurant, 1925/1926. gelatin print.
**23 x 28cm. SZ.2187.**

**35.** Meeting of the 1931/1932 Council of the Pharmaceutical Society, at 17 Bloomsbury Square, London. Those attending included the president, A.R. Melhuish, the Secretary, H. Linstead, J. Keall, E. Saville-Peck, A. Freke, T. Marns, J. Jack, T. Guthrie, and F. Browne. gelatin print.
**15 x 21cm. SZ.2189.**

**36.** Council of the Pharmaceutical Society, 17 Bloomsbury Square, London, 1975. gelatin print.
**20 x 25cm. SZ.2196.**

**37.** The Bristol Pharmaceutical Association, c.1890. albumen print.
**19 x 22cm (mounted). SZ.927.**

**38.** Jacob Bell memorial scholar, Charles Umney, 1862. albumen print, *carte-de-visite*.
**9 x 5.5cm (mounted in album). SZ.351.**

**39.** Jacob Bell memorial scholar, Alfred Neobard Palmer, 1867. albumen print, *carte-de-visite*.
**9 x 5.5cm (mounted in album). SZ.360.**

**40.** Jacob Bell memorial scholar, Henry George Greenish, 1875. albumen print, *carte-de-visite*.
**9 x 5.5cm (mounted in album). SZ.374.**

**41.** Jacob Bell memorial scholar, John Leaver West, 1875. albumen print, *carte-de-visite*.
**9 x 5.5cm (mounted in album). SZ.375.**

**42.** Jacob Bell memorial scholar, Joyce M. Carr, 1921. gelatin print, postcard.
**9 x 5.5cm (mounted in album). SZ.662.**

**43.** Harriett M. Bensley, annuitant of Pharmaceutical Society Benevolent Fund in 1891, taken c.1860. albumen print, *carte-de-visite*.
**10.4 x 6.3cm (mounted). SZ.1287.**

**44.** R. Mowbray, annuitant of Pharmaceutical Society Benevolent Fund in 1891, c.1891. gelatin print, *carte-de-visite:* J. Simpson, 7 Sneyd Street, Tunstall.
**9.5 x 6cm (mounted). SZ.1348.**

**45.** G. Foster, annuitant of Pharmaceutical Society Benevolent Fund in 1897, c.1860. albumen print, *carte-de-visite:* H. Hutching's Photographic Rooms, Hampstead Heath, London.
**9 x 5.5cm (mounted). SZ.1369.**

**46.** "The Last Watch of Hero": Professors Attfield, Redwood, and Bentley, c.1881-1887. photogravure.
**15 x 18cm (mounted). SZ.3096.**

**47.** Pharmaceutical Society board of examiners for Scotland, Scottish Branch, York Place, Edinburgh, including: G. Perrins, T. Wilson, J. Carruthers, Professor Sir W. Wright Smith, M. Morrison, J. Keall president of the Pharmaceutical Society, and the chairman J.H. Ramsay, 1933. gelatin print: J.C.H. Balmain, Edinburgh.
**23.5 x 29.5cm (mounted). SZ.923.**

**48.** Chemical laboratory, third floor, 17 Bloomsbury Square, including the Bell Scholars, Fraser McDiarmid and R. Wynn Charles Pierce, and the senior demonstrator, 1883/4. albumen print: Martin & Sallnow, 416 Strand, London WC.
**15.5 x 21cm (mounted). SZ.2.**

**49.** The "major chemical laboratory", third floor, 17 Bloomsbury Square, 1883/4. albumen print: Martin & Sallnow, 416 Strand, London WC.
**15.5 x 21cm (mounted). SZ. 1.**

**50.** The laboratory steward's bench in the major chemical laboratory, third floor, 17 Bloomsbury Square, 1883/4. albumen print: Martin & Sallnow, 416 Strand, London WC.
**15 x 20.5cm (mounted). SZ.3.**

**51.** The "chemical laboratory", third floor, 17 Bloomsbury Square, 1892. gelatin print.
**24 x 29.5cm (mounted). SZ.4.**

**52.** The old still in the chemistry laboratory with the laboratory assistant H. Caines, 17 Bloomsbury Square, c.1901. gelatin print: T.E. Wallis.
**10 x 7.5cm (mounted in album). SZ.1176.**

**53.** T.E. Wallis in the chemistry laboratory at 17 Bloomsbury Square, 1898. gelatin print.
**7.9 x 10.25cm (mounted). SZ.1256.**

**54.** A botanical ramble by the School on Hayes Common led by Professor H.G. Greenish, 1921. gelatin print: T. E. Wallis.
**4 x 7cm (mounted in album). SZ.1258.**

**55.** "Laboratory for applied pharmaceutics showing layout with two copper stills, steam heated pan etc.", 17 Bloomsbury Square, c.1901-1904. gelatin print: T.E. Wallis.
**11.5 x 15.5cm (mounted in album). SZ.1227.**

**56.** The lecture theatre of the School of Pharmacy, 17 Bloomsbury Square, 1892. gelatin print.
**29.5 x 24.5cm (mounted). SZ.7.**

**57.** The lecture theatre of the School of Pharmacy with Professor Greenish speaking, 1931. gelatin print.
**15.5 x 21cm. SZ.1782.**

**58.** The modernised lecture theatre at the School of Pharmacy, with W.H. Linnell demonstrating, c.1931. gelatin print.
**15 x 21cm. SZ.1747.**

**59.** Group photograph of the School of Pharmacy football team, Bloomsbury Square, 1911/1912. gelatin print.
**24 x 28cm (mounted). SZ.2209.**

**60.** Group photograph of the School of Pharmacy hockey team, Bloomsbury Square, including: C.W. Robinson, E.R. Withell, 1934/1935. gelatin print: H. Flett & Co. (H. Flett & A.F. Stevens), 118/119 Cheapside, London EC2.
**15 x 21cm. SZ.2068.**

**61.** Group photograph of students and staff of the School of Pharmacy, 17 Bloomsbury Square, c.1907. gelatin print: H. Flett, 119 Cheapside, London EC.
**24 x 29cm (mounted). SZ.3040.**

**62.** Group photograph of students and staff of the School of Pharmacy, including: T.E. Wallis, Professor Henry Greenish, H. Linstead, Marriot, Wolfitt, Brasher, Squire, Lester, Sumner, Day-Lewis, Short, Arkel, and Dyer, 1921/1922. gelatin print.
**24.4 x 29.5cm (mounted). SZ.2168.**

**63.** The students peculiar ritual leg-examination at the School of Pharmacy, 17 Bloomsbury Square, 1963/1964. gelatin print.
**13 x 18cm. SZ.2101.**

**64.** The School of Pharmacy at Brunswick Square, originally intended to be the new headquarters of the Pharmaceutical Society, 1950s. gelatin print, postcard.
**ll x 16cm. SZ.5368.**

**65.** The Metropolitan College of Pharmacy, 160/162 Kennington Park Road, London, c.1905. gelatin print: H. Teak, 12 Clapham Road, London SW.
**22 x 28cm (mounted). SZ.2000.**

**66.** *Argus* day, at the South London School of Pharmacy, 1940. gelatin print: S.J. Turner.
**4.5 x 5.5cm (mounted in album). SZ.1478.**

**67.** Group photograph of Muter's College (South London School of Pharmacy), 325 Kennington Road, London, with John Muter seated in the centre, 1896. gelatin print.
**24 x 30cm. SZ.2079.**

**68.** The annual dinner of the South of England College of Pharmacy, The Holborn Restaurant, London, 9 June 1910. gelatin print: Fradelle & Young, 283 Regent Street, London.
**22 x 35cm (mounted). SZ.2061.**

**69.** The Manchester School of Pharmacy, c.l900. gelatin print: J. Cleworth, Chemist & Photographer, 56 Ducie Street, Manchester.
**10.5 x 15.5cm (mounted). SZ.2042.**

**70.** Riverboat excursion, Henley-on-Thames, International Pharmacy Congress, London, 1881. gelatin copy print.
**20 x 25cm. SZ.298.**

**71.** Delegates to the Fifth International Congress of Military Medicine, seated in Bloomsbury Square, London 10 May, 1929. gelatin print: H. Flett & Co., 119 Cheapside, London EC2.
**24.5 x 30cm. SZ.3090.**

**72.** Members of the Bureau, including Sir Hugh Linstead, Dr E. Höst (president), and Dr H. Birza (general secretary) at the Ordre National des Pharmaciens, International Pharmaceutical Federation, Paris, 1953. gelatin print.
**23.2 x 10cm (mounted). SZ.4030.**

**73.** The British Pharmaceutical Conference, Dundee, visit to Craighall, Blairgowrie, Perth, 1867. Delegates include Professor Bentley, Professor Attfield, Henry Deane, and Albert E. Ebert of Chicago, 5 September 1867. albumen print: Abbot, Dundee.
**18 x 24cm (mounted). SZ.2044.**

**74.** British Pharmaceutical Conference, Bristol, 1903. The visit to Tintern Abbey, Monmouthshire, 30 July 1903. gelatin print.
**26 x 36cm (mounted). SZ.2047.**

**75.** British Pharmaceutical Conference, Newcastle-upon-Tyne, group photograph taken at Jesmond Dene July 27 1909. gelatin print: Thompson & Lee, Newcastle-on-Tyne.
**24 x 33cm. SZ.2049.**

**76.** British Pharmaceutical Conference, Dublin, 31 July 1901. gelatin print: Lafayette, Dublin.
**26 x 34.5cm (mounted). SZ.2046.**

**77.** British Pharmaceutical Conference, visit to the Roman Baths, 1924. gelatin print: probably by J. Cleworth.
**12 x 17cm. SZ.2043.**

**78.** British Pharmaceutical Conference, Scarborough Spa, Yorkshire, 15 June 1921. gelatin print: H. L. Ke[-]le, 18 Ramshill Road, Scarborough, Yorks.
**29 x 43cm. SZ.2261.**

**79.** "At Tuesday's Luncheon", the BPC Ex-Servicemen's Table, British Pharmaceutical Conference, Liverpool, 27 July 1937. gelatin print.
**12.3 x 19.8cm (mounted). SZ.3900.**

**80.** "Visitors on Board a Liner, Miss Smail with Mr and Mrs Clubb". British Pharmaceutical Conference visit to Birkenhead. 1937. gelatin print.
**12.9 x 11.25cm (mounted). SZ.3894.**

**81.** The Peebles Excursion "Hurrying for the bus", British Pharmaceutical Conference, Edinburgh, 1938. gelatin print.
**13.4 x 12.3cm (mounted). SZ.3602.**

**82.** "The Excursion down the Clyde. A group of young hospital pharmacists". British Pharmaceutical Conference, Edinburgh, September 1950. gelatin print.
**14.9 x 18.2cm (mounted). SZ.3585.**

**83.** "The River Excursion from Westminster to Greenwich Pier. The second boat arriving at Greenwich Pier". British Pharmaceutical Conference, London, 3 September 1953. gelatin print.
**6.3 x 15.3cm (mounted). SZ.3755.**

**84.** "The River Excursion from Westminster to Greenwich Pier. The Chairman of the Conference with his mother and sister". British Pharmaceutical Conference, London, National Maritime Museum, 2 September 1953. gelatin print.
**9.9 x 15.3cm (mounted). SZ.3756.**

**85.** John Bell & Co. Chemists, 338 Oxford Street, London, c. 1870. albumen print: photographer unknown, but probably S.A. Walker.
**17 x 10cm (mounted). SZ.999.**

**86.** The front-shop of John Bell & Co. as redesigned by Theophilus Redwood in 1824, c.l900. modern print from original gelatin dry plate.
**12 x 16.4cm. SZ.5999.**

**87.** John Bell & Co., 338 Oxford Street, London Wl, 1871. Thomas Hyde Hills is centre left. albumen print from wet collodion negative: S.A. Walker, 64 Margaret Street, Cavendish Square, London.
**15 x 20cm (mounted). SZ 233.**

**88.** John Bell & Co., 338 Oxford Street, London Wl, 1871. albumen print from wet collodion negative: S.A. Walker, 64 Margaret Street, Cavendish Square, London.
**15 x 20cm (mounted). SZ.234.**

**89.** The exterior of the old building of Allen & Hanbury's pharmacy, 2 Plough Court, London, after the modernisations of 1856 and before its demolition in 1873. The new premises were destroyed by bombing in 1940. gelatin copy print.
**21 x 25cm. SZ.5603.**

**90.** The shopfront of William Hooper & Co., 24 Russell Street, Covent Garden, London, c.l900. gelatin print.
**24 x 29cm. SZ.6001.**

**91.** The laboratory of William Hooper & Co., 24 Russell Street, Covent Garden, London, c.1908. toned gelatin print: Ball, 11 Wilton Road, Victoria Station, London SW.
**24.5 x 29.5cm. (mounted). SZ.2250.**

**92.** Detail of the much-repaired 60 gallon still at 24 Russell Street, c.l900. gelatin print.
**25.5 x 20.5cm. SZ.2712.**

**93.** The small dispensary of T. Cox at 35 Trumpington Street, Cambridge, before 1876. gelatin copy print.
**14 x 11cm. SZ.3072.**

**94.** A. Deck Chymist, 9 King's Parade, Cambridge, 1872. albumen print, *carte-de-visite:* W.I. Pashler.
**9.5 x 5.5cm (mounted). SZ.3058.**

**95.** Deck Pharmaceutical Chymist, 9 King's Parade, Cambridge, c.1899. gelatin print, postcard.
**14 x 9cm. SZ.3059.**

**96.** G. Peck & Son, Chemists, 9 King's Parade, Cambridge, 1920s. gelatin print.
**11 x 14cm. SZ.3070.**

**97.** G. Peck, 30 Trumpington Street, Cambridge, c.1890. gelatin print.
**11 x 13cm. SZ.3071.**

**98.** The exterior of Heppel & Co., 164 Piccadilly, London, 1912. gelatin print: John H. Avery & Co., 40 Hillmarton Road, London, N.
**24.5 x 29.5cm (mounted in album). SZ. 1044.**

**99.** The dispensing area of Heppel & Co., 164 Piccadilly, London, 1912. gelatin print: John H. Avery & Co., 40 Hillmarton Road, London, N.
**24.5 x 29.5cm (mounted in album). SZ.1046.**

**100.** Heppel & Co., 164 Piccadilly, London, 1912. gelatin print: John H. Avery & Co., 40 Hillmarton Road, London, N.
**24.5 x 29.5cm (mounted in album). SZ.1047.**

**101.** Heppel & Co. Chemists, 77-78 Strand, London, 1912 . gelatin print: John H. Avery & Co., 40 Hillmarton Road, London, N.
**24.5 x 29.5cm (mounted in album). SZ.1041.**

**102.** Heppel & Co. Chemists, Hotel Cecil Buildings, 77-78 Strand, London, 1912. gelatin print: John H. Avery & Co., 40 Hillmarton Road, London, N.
**24.5 x 29.5cm (mounted in album). SZ.1042.**

**103.** Heppel & Co. Chemists, Hotel Cecil Buildings, 77-78 Strand, London, 1912. gelatin print: John H . Avery & Co., 40 Hillmarton Road, London, N.
**24.5 x 29.5cm (mounted in album). SZ.1043.**

**104.** Exterior of Heppel & Co. Pharmacie Française, 35 Haymarket, London, 1912. gelatin print: John H. Avery & Co., 40 Hillmarton Road, London, N.
**24.5 x 29.5cm (mounted in album). SZ.1048.**

**105.** Interior of Heppel & Co. Pharmacie Française, 35 Haymarket, London, 1912. gelatin print: John H. Avery & Co., 40 Hillmarton Road, London, N.
**24.5 x 29.5cm (mounted in album). SZ.1049.**

**106.** Exterior of Heppel & Co., 4 St Michaels Alley, 1912. Heppel's were agents for Wrigley's "Pepsin" gum. gelatin print: John H. Avery & Co., 40 Hillmarton Road, London, N.
**24.5 x 29.5cm (mounted in album). SZ.1050.**

**107.** Interior of Heppel & Co., 4 St Michaels Alley, 1912. gelatin print: John H. Avery & Co., 40 Hillmarton Road, London, N.
**24.5 x 29.5cm (mounted in album). SZ.1051.**

**108.** Cross Street and Essex Road corner, Islington, London, opposite to the Wallis pharmacy, 1903. gelatin print: T.E. Wallis.
**11.5 X 15.5cm. SZ.1183.**

**109.** "Charlie's photo of father's shop". Wallis Pharmaceutical Chemist patent medicine & drug stores, 78 Essex Road, Islington. The premises of J.T.W. Wallis PhC, 1895. gelatin print: C.D. Wallis.
**10.7 x 8cm. SZ 1276.**

**110.** 78 Essex Road counter, the interior of Wallis Pharmaceutical Chemist patent medicine & drug stores, 1902. gelatin print: T.E. Wallis.
**11.5 x 15.5cm. SZ.1204.**

**111.** Above the shop at 78 Essex Road, 1902. gelatin print: T.E. Wallis.
**11.5 x 15.5cm. SZ.1201.**

**112.** An early multiple store: Wride & Co., 34 High Street, Shirley, Hampshire, c.1880-1890. albumen print.
**11 x 16cm. SZ.195.**

**113.** The original premises of Wride & Co., at 1-2 The Strand, East Street, Southampton prior to demolition in 1929. gelatin print.
**9 x 13cm. SZ.194.**

**114.** "Averill's old shop". Boots was the prime example of the cash chemist. Boots dispensing chemists, 10-11 Market Square, Stafford, 1950s. gelatin print.
**30 x 25cm. SZ.2167.**

**115.** Deane & Co. dispensing chemists, 17 The Pavement, Clapham, London, October 1953. gelatin print.
**22 x 17cm (mounted). SZ.138.**

**116.** Beken & Son Chemists, Cowes, Isle of Wight, c.1900. Beken specialised in maritime photography. gelatin print.
**21 x 27cm. SZ.137.**

**117.** James Stevens with his daughter, probably on the opening of his pharmacy, 6 High Street, New Brompton (Gillingham), 1872. albumen print.
**9.8 x 7.2cm (mounted). SZ.6100.**

**118.** Robert E. Price Dispensing Chemist, 72 High Street, Rhyl, 1909. gelatin print, postcard.
**14 x 9cm. SZ.3068.**

**119.** Pharmacy in Enfield Town: Successor to John Tuff, Enfield, Middlesex, c.1898-1918. gelatin print.
**38 x 27cm. SZ.85.**

**120.** Boilerhouse and laboratory in the pharmacy of Nathaniel Smith, a founder member of the Society. This pharmacy was established by Lea & Perrins, of the "Worcestershire" sauce. 373 High Street, Cheltenham, Gloucester, c.1900. platinum print.
**18.5 x 22.5cm (mounted). SZ.244.**

**121.** The Penton Pharmacy, London, c.1930. gelatin print.
**16 x 21cm. SZ.167.**

**122.** Leonard's Pharmacy, London, c.1930. gelatin print.
**21 x 16cm. SZ.131.**

**123.** Retail establishments in Leeds: A paste-up montage of photographs to illustrate an article on the 1934 British Pharmaceutical Conference in *The Pharmaceutical Journal,* including: Harold Haw MPS, Chemist; J.R. Bentley & Son, est.130 years; Bells old pharmacy; A.L. Peters, MPS Dispensing Chemist; F.C. Long, Headingly Pharmacy, Optician, Pharmaceutical Chemist; R. Milestone MPS Dispensing Chemist; Armitage MPS Pharmaceutical Chemist, 114 Armley Grove Place, Leeds, 1934. gelatin print.

**30 x 37cm. SZ.2255,**
**13 x 17cm. SZ.2256,**
**14 x 13cm. SZ.2257,**
**15.5 x 10.5cm. SZ.2258,**
**14 x 15cm. SZ.2259,**
**14 x 15cm. SZ.2260 (mounted together).**
**SZ.2255-2260.**

**124.** The exterior of T. & F. J. Taylor Pharmacists, 36 High Street, Newport Pagnell, Buckinghamshire, decorated for the Royal jubilee of 1935. gelatin print.
**6 x 8cm. SZ.3081.**

**125.** "The manner in which two existing shopfronts have been linked": The pharmacy of E.T.S. Steel, MPS, chemist, 58-59 East Street, Southampton, modernised in the 1930s, "bronze and marble" style, 1939. gelatin print.
**15 x 21cm. SZ.209.**

**126.** Claude Benton Ltd., Norwich, c.1950. gelatin print: A.J. Seymour & Co., 18a Prince of Wales Road, Norwich.
**17.5 x 24cm. SZ.108.**

**127.** The interior of the new premises of Gordon Smith, MPS, dispensing chemist of Ashley Road, Hale, Cheshire, 1938. gelatin print: S. Bale, 13 Union Court, Liverpool 2.
**29 x 24cm. SZ.97.**

**128.** The new eye-test room and equipment at Forster, Chemist Optician, 11 Faircross Parade, New Barking, Essex, 1930s. gelatin print.
**17.5 x 13cm. (mounted). SZ.82.**

**129.** One of the series of exteriors of traditional pharmacies collected by the History of Pharmacy Committee: S.N. White, The Pharmacy, Topsham, Devon, established in 1823. c.1953. gelatin print.
**16 x 20cm (mounted). SZ.146.**

**130.** The exterior of G. R. Oke, 14 Market Place, Aylsham, Norfolk, 1953. gelatin print.
**20 x 15cm. SZ.3066.**

**131.** "The Pharmacist in retail practice". The interior of the pharmacy of R. J. Mellowes, 20 Bush Hill Parade, Enfield, Middlesex, 1959. gelatin print.
**20 x 24cm. SZ.103.**

**132.** The pharmacy department, St George's Hospital, London, c.1950. gelatin print.
**14.5 x 21cm. SZ.255.**

**133.** "The Pharmacist in hospital: the dispensary", St Bartholomew's Hospital, London, 1959. gelatin print.
**20 x 24cm. SZ.104.**

**134.** The staff of Rankin & Co. Druggists, 7 King Street, Kilmarnock, c.1890. gelatin print.
**15 x 20.5cm. SZ.712.**

**135.** The staff of Taylors' Drug Co. Ltd., 16 Beulah Street to 54 Station Parade, Harrogate, c.1900. Charles H. White M.P.S. (1880-1961) seated centre. gelatin print
**15 x 21cm (mounted). SZ.715.**

**136.** The Payne family, Newcastle-upon-Tyne, Northumberland, 1890s. gelatin print.
**10.5 x 15.5cm (mounted). SZ.1494.**

**137.** John Bell, Hills & Lucas Ltd., staff outing, 29 September 1919. gelatin print: G.E. Boxall, Parisian School of Photography, 246 Old Kent Road, London.
**15 x 20.5cm (mounted). SZ.1039.**

**138.** John Bell, Hills & Lucas Ltd., staff outing, 1919 gelatin print: G.E. Boxall, Parisian School of Photography, 246 Old Kent Road, London.
**15 x 20.5cm (mounted). SZ.1040.**

**139.** Mrs Attfield at home, Ashlands, Watford, Hertfordshire, 10 July 1897. toned gelatin print: W. Coles, 60 Queens Road, Watford.
**25 x 36cm (mounted). SZ.2264.**

**140.** Maw challenge shield competition, New Barnet, 1925. gelatin print.
**21.55 x 15cm. (mounted in album). SZ.1651.**

**141.** Maw challenge shield competition, New Barnet, 1925. gelatin print.
**8 x 12cm (mounted in album). SZ.l910.**

**142.** Maw challenge shield competition, New Barnet, 1923. gelatin print.
**16 x 20.5cm (mounted in album). SZ.1605.**

**143.** View of San Carlos cinchona plantation with the proprietor Señor Don Manuel Calderon, Bolivia, 20 December 1882. albumen print: photographer unknown, possibly Charles Ledger.
**18 x 23cm. SZ.1802.**

**144.** View of cinchona plants in the propagating house at the Government gardens Ootacamund, Madras, India, 9 September 1861. albumen print.
**18 x 23cm. SZ.1803.**

**145.** Production of smoking opium at the Government Monopoly Factory, Hong Kong, 1915. Showing the separated piths and skins of the opened opium balls. gelatin print: H. Alan Taylor.
**8.5 x 10.5cm. SZ.2567.**

**146.** Exterior of the rubber warehouse and facilities of the Argos Steamship Co., London & Bremen Line, St Katherine's docks, with moored freighter, c.1910. toned gelatin print: Tella Camera Co., 68 High Holborn, London WC.
**24 x 29cm. SZ.344.**

**147.** Interior of the rubber vaults, St Katherine's docks, London, c.1910. toned gelatin print: Tella Camera Co., 68 High Holborn, London WC.
**24 x 29cm. SZ.347.**

**148.** "Antigas" work. Fitting-up box-respirator gas masks at the Oxford Works, Tower Bridge Road, c.1917/1918. gelatin print: John H. Avery & Co., Commercial Photographers, 40 Hillmarton Road, London, N.
**23.5 x 28cm (mounted). SZ.2703.**

**149.** Printing and labelling room, 1933. gelatin print: John H. Avery & Co., Publicity Photographers, 426 Camden Road, N7.
**24 x 28.5cm (mounted). SZ.4611.**

**150.** Manufacturing plant, John Bell, Hills & Lucas, 1933. gelatin print: John H. Avery & Co., Publicity Photographers, 426 Camden Road, N7.
**24 x 28.5cm (mounted). SZ.4612.**

**151.** Steedman's stall at a baby show, Derby, c.l900. gelatin print: Gibson & Sons, St Peter's Street, Derby.
**11 x 15cm (mounted). SZ.311.**

**152.** Delivery van in Steedman's livery. The bodywork of 1913 adapted to a Beardmore chassis, 1922. gelatin print.
**15 x 20.5cm. SZ.300.**

**153.** A Steedman's Morris delivery van, Walworth, Surrey, November 1956. gelatin print: J. Schafer.
**16 x 21cm. SZ.305.**

## Note to the Illustrations Index

The original titles of photographs and details are indicated where known.

Photographers names and addresses follow process information.

Dimensions are given in centimetres for the image area only, height preceding width, excluding any mounts.

# PHOTOGRAPHER INDEX

**Plate No.**

Abbot,
Dundee, 73

John H. Avery & Co.,
40 Hillmarton Road, London, N, 98-107

John H. Avery & Co.,
Commercial Photographers,
40 Hillmarton Road, London, N, 148

John H. Avery & Co.,
Publicity Photographers,
426 Camden Road, N7, 149, 150

S. Bale,
13 Union Court, Liverpool, 2, 127

Ball,
11 Wilton Road, Victoria Station,
London SW, 91

J.C.H. Balmain,
Edinburgh, 47

Barrauds Ltd.,
263 Oxford Street W.
(Regent Circus), London, 18

G.E. Boxall,
Parisian School of Photography,
246 Old Kent Road, London, 137, 138

J. Cleworth,
Chemist & Photographer,
56 Ducie Street, Manchester, 69

J. Cleworth (?), 77

W. Coles,
60 Queens Road, Watford, 139

R.B. Fleming & Co., 10, 15, 17

H. Flett & Co.
(H. Flett & A.F. Stevens),
118/119 Cheapside, London EC2, 60

H. Flett,
119 Cheapside, London EC, 61

H. Flett & Co.,
119 Cheapside, London EC2, 71

Fradelle & Young,
283 Regent Street, London, 68

Gibson & Sons,
St Peter's Street, Derby, 151

Horne & Thornthwaite,
121, 122, 123, Newgate Street,
London, 23

H. Hutching's
Photographic Rooms,
Hampstead Heath, London, 45

H. L. Ke[-]lle,
18 Ramshill Road, Scarborough,
Yorks, 78

Lafayette,
Dublin, 76

Charles Ledger (?), 143

Martin & Sallnow,
416 Strand, London WC, 3, 5, 11, 48, 49, 50

Martin & Sallnow (?), 7, 9

Maull & Co.,
62 Cheapside EC,
187 Piccadilly & Tavistock House,
London, 24, 25, 26, 28, 29, 30

Maull & Co.,
187a Piccadilly W,
62 Cheapside EC, Tavistock House,
Fulham Road, London, 21

Maull & Co.,
187a Piccadilly &
62 Cheapside, London, 33

Maull & Fox,
187a Piccadilly, London, 32

J.E. Mayall,
224 Regent Street,
Daguerreotype Institution,
433 West Strand, 19

Miles & Kaye Ltd.,
100 Southampton Row,
High Holborn, London WCl, 4

Nadar,
photographie du Grand Hotel,
35 Boulevart des Capucines,
Paris, 27

W.I. Pashler, 94

John T. Sandell (?), 6

J. Schafer, 153

A.J. Seymour & Co.,
18a Prince of Wales Road,
Norwich, 126

J. Simpson,
7 Sneyd Street, Tunstall, 44

Sir Joseph Wilson Swan (?), 1

H. Alan Taylor, 145

H. Teak,
12 Clapham Road, London SW, 65

Tella Camera Co.,
68 High Holborn, London WC, 146-147

Thompson & Lee,
Newcastle-on-Tyne, 75

The "Topical" Press Agency Ltd.,
10 & 11 Red Lion Court,
Fleet Street, London EC4, 16

S.J. Turner, 66

S.A. Walker,
64 Margaret Street,
Cavendish Square, London, 87, 88

S.A. Walker (?), 85

W. Walker & Sons,
64 Margaret Street,
Cavendish Square, London, 20, 22

C.D. Wallis, 109

T.E. Wallis, 52, 54, 55, 108, 110, 111

## Note to sources and further reading

The quoted comments in the biographical sketches are mostly taken from the generally anonymous obituary notices published in *The Pharmaceutical Journal,* 1841-, and *The Chemist and Druggist,* 1861-.

There is an extensive literature concerning the history of photography, but Helmut and Alison Gernsheim, *The History of Photography,* London, Oxford University Press, 1969, remains one of the best general introductions to the subject.

For dating photographs two useful works are: Madeleine Ginsburg, *Victorian Dress in Photographs,* London, Batsford, 1988, and Michael Pritchard, *A Directory of London Photographers 1841-1908,* Watford, ALLM Books, 1986. The Royal Photographic Society has in addition published several regional directories of early photographers.